THE CHRONIC ILLNESS
TRAJECTORY FRAMEWORK

The Corbin and Strauss Nursing Model

Editor

Pierre Woog, Ph.D., one of the founding editors of *Scholarly Inquiry for Nursing Practice,* is professor of Human Service Studies at Adelphi University as well as Professor of Education and Professor of Nursing. Formerly he was the Founding Dean of Adelphi School of Education. He has extensive experience in graduate teaching and has consulted, authored articles and books, and made presentations in the fields of Education, Nursing, Mental Health, Evaluation, Research Methodology, and Psychometrics. Currently he spends some time as the occasional essayist for the journal *Evaluation and Health Professions.*

Editors of *Scholarly Inquiry for Nursing Practice*

THE CHRONIC ILLNESS TRAJECTORY FRAMEWORK

The Corbin and Strauss Nursing Model

Pierre Woog
Editor

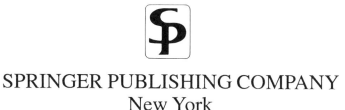

SPRINGER PUBLISHING COMPANY
New York

Copyright © 1992 by Springer Publishing Company, Inc.

Springer Publishing Company, Inc.
536 Broadway
New York, NY 10012

    93 94 95 96 / 5 4 3 2

Library of Congress Cataloging in Publication Data

The Chronic illness trajectory framework: the Corbin and Strauss
    nursing model / Pierre Woog, editor.
            p.   cm.
            Includes bibliographical references.
            ISBN 0-8261-8000-0
            1. Chronic disease—nursing. I. Woog, Pierre.
            [DNLM: 1. Chronic disease—nursing 2. Models, Nursing.
    WY 152 C5576]
    RT120.C45C5 1992
    610.73—dc20
    DNLM/DLC
    for Library of Congress   91-5198

Printed in the United States of America

Contents

Contributors

Juliet Corbin, R.N., D.N.Sc., is associated with both San Jose State University and the University of California at San Francisco as a lecturer and research associate. She has written extensively in the areas of nursing care, health care systems, and the flow of work in hospitals. With Anselm Strauss, she has recently authored the highly praised Sage book, *Basics of Qualitative Research.*

Diane Scott Dorsett, R.N., Ph.D., F.A.A.N., is the founder and currently Director of Comprehensive Support Services for Persons with Cancer, and conducts a private practice in San Francisco, CA. She is adjunct Associate Clinical Professor, University of California School of Nursing, Department of Physiological Nursing, San Francisco, and Attending Scientist, the Medical Research Institute, an independent research facility affiliated with Pacific Presbyterian Medical Center, San Francisco. She was formerly Nurse Scientist at Memorial Sloan-Kettering Cancer Center, New York, and a Robert Wood Johnson Clinical Nurse Scholar at the University of California at San Francisco.

Mary Hawthorne, Ph.D., R.N., is an assistant professor at Duke University. She has written and presented in the areas of coronary artery surgery recovery and critical care. Currently, her special area of interest is the recovery of women after cardiac arrest.

Kathleen Nokes, Ph.D., R.N., is an Assistant Professor at Hunter College and the project director of a Department of Health and Human Services Training Grant to create a subspecialization in the nursing care of persons with HIV/AIDS. She has written and presented in the areas of AIDS and HIV as related to counseling, community-based care, and legal, moral, and ethical issues.

Marilyn Rawnsley, D.N.S.C., R.N., C.S., is a Professor of Nursing at Teachers College, Columbia University, and an ANA-certified clinical specialist in psychiatric mental health nursing. She has extensive experience in graduate teaching, research, and clinical consulting, and has written books, articles, and presentations in the field of mental health and issues pertaining to knowledge development in nursing.

Suzanne Smeltzer, R.N., C., Ed.D., is an associate professor and nurse researcher at the Department of Nursing, College of Allied Health Sciences of Thomas Jefferson University in Philadelphia. She has published numerous articles and conducted sponsored research about multiple sclerosis.

Anselm Strauss, Ph.D., is Professor Emeritus of the University of California at San Francisco. He is a world-renowned sociologist, perhaps best known for "grounded theory," and has been a visiting professor from the University of Cambridge to the University of Adelaide. He has written extensively about qualitative and historical methodology and the sociologies of health and illness and of work and the professions.

Elizabeth Walker, D.N.Sc., R.N., is a certified diabetes educator, Assistant Professor of Epidemiology and Social Medicine at The Albert Einstein College of Medicine and a nurse researcher at the Diabetes Research and Training Center at Albert Einstein. She is also one of the research nurses in the Diabetes Control and Complications Trial, the nationwide DCCT Study. Walker has worked in both inpatient and outpatient settings as an educator and nurse clinician and is a consultant for quality assurance issues related to blood glucose monitoring.

Introduction

This book came about as a special issue of the journal *Scholarly Inquiry for Nursing Practice*. It describes Corbin and Strauss' nursing model for chronic illness management, and reactions to it by six nurses expert in the "realities" of helping people with cancer, cardiac conditions, mental illness, diabetes, multiple sclerosis, and HIV/AIDS. The editors and publisher felt that this important material should reach the general nursing community at large beyond the researchers and theorists who make up our journal readership. This book serves that purpose. We believe that this book can engender a significant change in how we regard chronic disease and the betterment of health.

To best explicate the work of Corbin and Strauss, six nurse researchers, each expert in a chronic disease, were asked to respond to Chapter 1, by Corbin and Strauss. What would such a model mean within their work? We then asked Corbin and Strauss to respond to these six experts. This introduction highlights the various articles and analyzes the possible strengths of the model and concerns about it within each disease entity and across entities. It will finish with a consideration, perhaps a meditation, upon the issues raised.

The Corbin and Strauss chapter, "A Nursing Model for Chronic Illness Management Based Upon the Trajectory Framework," presents a view of chronic illness with eight phases from pretrajectory to dying, with each possessing the possibilities of reversals, plateaus, and upward and/or downward movement. This trajectory is mediated by personal biographies and characteristics, the "vision of the course," influential conditions comprised of resources embedded within the culture in its social, political, and economic manifestations and the management schema that shape the illness on the part of the patient, caretakers, loved ones, and health providers. It is a dynamic model, for there is much uncertainty and details cannot be fully determined in advance.

It is an important model because it can enable us to better conceptualize the course of illness and, as such, we can envision and create better policy, we can conduct research to better understand the processes, and, with this understanding, we can give better care. Finally, the model centers on the patient and affirms that his/her perceptions and beliefs about what is and may be happening to him/her are paramount to predicting the nature of the trajectory. Thus, the model is rich. It is client focused, conceptually sophisticated. It engenders research, care plans, and policy changes which improve health.

Diane Scott Dorsett's "The Trajectory of Cancer Recovery" responds to Corbin and Strauss by making a case for a recovery model. Because she feels that cancer is a chronic disease characterized by episodes, acute morbidities, more prolonged remissions and, in many cases, cure, she believes the trajectory model condenses the cancer experience into a time warp of symptom-driven illness mediated by medical treatments until death occurs. She believes that a recovery model is more appropriate because it focuses upon absorption, assimilation, and accommodation to the disease process, and is, as such, user friendly. Recovery is characterized by renewal and recuperation, which is collaborative and cooperative, rather than focused on compliance.

Mary Hawthorne's "Using the Trajectory Framework: Reconceptualizing Cardiac Illness" makes the following observations about cardiac illness that may be particular to this disease entity.

- The patient first becomes aware of hypertension.
- An increasing number of patients survive myocardial infarction, thus morbidity may be more central than death or care and is often confounded by aging.
- There is an emerging population of chronically critically ill.
- Powerful technology reinforces the medical (cure) paradigm of acute illness.

She views the trajectory model as particularly potent in that there are gender trajectory differences in biographies, timing and demands on the patient. Trajectory can identify consistent caregivers rather than fragmented episode-directed care, and trajectory forces future orientation with anticipated potential problems and planned behavioral reductions of risk behaviors.

Kathleen Nokes, in "Applying the Chronic Illness Trajectory Model to HIV/ AIDS," makes important contributions to the discussion. First, the inclusion of HIV/AIDS from the perspective of chronic disease is most important. As we as a culture begin to better understand this disease and its chronic nature (the time from diagnosis to possible death keeps increasing), we will be better able to make intelligent policy decisions and render better long-term care. Second, Nokes focuses upon HIV/AIDS within the Corbin-Strauss model and makes the following important points.

The first phase has two, rather than one, crisis points: learning one is HIV positive and learning one shows symptoms of AIDS. Each has its own vision, i.e., aggressive action and hopelessness, respectively. Home care can be very problematic in that, given the problems of disclosure and discrimination, one may either not have a home or one must return to an alienated home. The need for health teaching to clarify misconceptions becomes paramount. Finally, Nokes points out that one can envision multiple disease trajectories, and accessibility and continuity as key to quality management.

Marilyn Rawnsley's "Chronic Mental Illness: The Timeless Trajectory" uses two case studies to examine the trajectory model and gives us a sense of poignancy. She believes that the model can revitalize psychiatric nursing and facilitate the nursing management aspect. Given the social stigma of mental disease and the impoverished and disorganized delivery system, this revitalization can be heralded.

Rawnsley makes some extremely worthy points in describing mental illness as a chronic disease. She states, for example, that the reciprocal effects of mental disorder on physical well-being, particularly adherence to a medical regimen, cannot be overemphasized. Furthermore, she characterizes the chronicity of major mental disorder as a timeless trajectory, seemingly without purpose, without progress, without resolution, and without end. As such, the focus of intervention is always short term and realistic; it is aimed at keeping the individual functioning in activities of daily living with minimal distress to self and others. The longer the span between crises, the more successful the intervention.

Suzanne Smeltzer's "Use of the Trajectory Model of Nursing in Multiple Sclerosis" focuses upon the waxing and waning of symptoms that make for wide variations among patients and the variation of symptoms, all of which make multiple sclerosis unpredictable in its overall course, in the occurrence of the next attack, in the type of symptoms that will predominate, in its eventual outcome, in its diagnosis, and in evaluating therapies. This unpredictability can, in many cases, offer hope. The trajectory model is helpful, for it can ensure a constancy of care and focus on establishing evaluation criteria upon the patient and the family. Finally, an abiding question for multiple sclerosis is the transition from illness to wellness.

Elizabeth Walker's "Shaping the Course of a Marathon: Using the Trajectory Framework for Diabetes Mellitus" reminds us of the necessity for day by day self-intervention and monitoring, the possible major behavioral changes that can occur, the complex regimens, and the variety of health providers, including, at least, the nurse specialist, the endocrinologist, and the dietician. All of these ongoing complexities and difficulties can result in patients' everchanging projection of visions of the trajectory. These can be further complicated by family histories that often provide conflicting messages about the trajectory projection for the person with diabetes. The daily struggle and ongoing changes for the diabetic person give the trajectory model a rich milieu for utilization.

A final commentary by Corbin and Strauss gives their reaction to the six response chapters. This discourse uncovers several important points which can be seen in two general ways. First, one can look at the six response chapters and see that all authors were able to conceptualize, internalize and apply the model to their particular disease entity. Thus, in the sense of Ernest House's "validity as argument," a great measure of the validity of the model is secured. Furthermore, there is great variation in the disease entities. We are faced with the notion of the chronically critically ill, we recognize the chronicity of AIDS, we struggle with the notions of timelessness and marathon, and we gird ourselves for the immense job that will be necessary politically, economically, and socially of giving the kind of care the trajectory model demands. Once more, we are reminded of the variations between and within illnesses and the courage of the patients and their families. Once more, we are reminded of the humanity of our efforts and we appreciate, one more time, the unrelenting change we face, whether in the waxing and waning of the disease entity or in the new miracles and/or new visions.

Second, we look at the trajectory model and raise questions. They are big questions and result from a big model. How do we reconcile trajectory and recovery? Diane Scott Dorsett raises the question, and Corbin and Strauss, in their commentary, soberly consider it. Trajectory, as defined by Corbin and Strauss, contains eight phases, the last being death. Death is the end oint. Furthermore, the word trajectory is defined, according to Webster's, as the curved path of something hurtling through space, especially that of a projectile from the time it leaves the muzzle of a gun. This conjures predictability and death, a martial vision. Yet Corbin and Strauss also tell us that trajectories are often uncertain and can only be graphed in retrospect. Scott Dorsett talks of survival, growth, change, and the user friendly.

Two thoughts come to mind. First, we all die. It may be that the illness trajectory is a metaphor for our lifespan, our mortality. The fact that we did survive, or even that we are cured from a disease, does not take us off the curved path. The experience of disease, however, as Corbin and Strauss point out in their commentary, impacts our biographies and our visions and, thus, our trajectories; it has consequences.

Second, we can see trajectory and recovery as a paradox, a yin and yang of health and illness, both valid, both irreconcilable, but merged. Both these visions, perhaps, must be held simultaneously. The literature of the helping professions can assist here. It is said that the best teachers simultaneously are with the student, a kind of Carl Rogers' "unconditional regard," subjective, intense, involved, and yet there is a third eye hovering, picking cues, in Schön's words, "reflecting in action," observing, hypothesizing, being objective. This paradox defines excellence in teaching. Perhaps, the trajectory image and the recovery image must also be held simultaneously by the nurse.

Another big question, not totally separate from the previous, is whether there is a cure, or "when is a chronic disease not chronic?" How long does one have to be symptom-free to say one no longer has X? A very close relative had a breast removed because of a cancer about 35 years ago. Is she in remission or is she cured? My 88-year-old father has a history of cardiac disease. He is active, engaged, and as critical in his judgment as ever. He takes medication, but does he suffer from chronic disease? A good friend, a nurse, has been symptom-free from multiple sclerosis for ten years. Does she suffer from a chronic disease? I had polio as a child. Do I have a chronic disease? These are fundamental questions, because how we answer them directly affects the trajectory model and within that context helps us define our visions and, subsequently, our biographies.

The Corbin and Strauss model of the trajectory of chronic illness, the six response chapters, and the commentary provide rich information and questions. They open new doors for research and are infused with the humanity of our calling. We hope that this book will bring forth more research, educational, and clinical efforts.

Pierre Woog, Ph.D.

A Nursing Model for Chronic Illness Management Based Upon the Trajectory Framework

Juliet M. Corbin, R.N., D.N.Sc.

Department of Nursing, San Jose State University,
San Jose, California,
School of Nursing, University of California, San Francisco

Anselm Strauss, Ph.D.

School of Nursing, University of California, San Francisco

The trajectory framework developed by Strauss and associates provides a conceptual basis for developing a nursing model that gives direction for practice, teaching, and research in the area of chronic illness. This paper presents an overview of the trajectory framework and shows how it can be used to generate such a nursing model.

The management of chronic conditions is more than just a matter of controlling symptoms, or living with disability, or adapting to the psychological and social changes that long-term incurable illness brings to the lives of afflicted individuals and their families. It is all of these and more. Therefore, any approach to the nursing care of the chronically ill and their families must be comprehensive and reflect the diversity, multiplicity, and complexity of the problems that chronic conditions can bring.

While a considerable body of nursing literature has accumulated in the area of chronic illness, much of it is illness specific (Cronin, 1986; Dunkel-Schetter, 1984; Lovejoy, 1986; O'Connor, 1983; Popkess-Vawter, 1983), is focused on specific management problems (Dai & Catanzaro, 1987; Dodd, 1984; Gillis, 1984), or examines the relationship between several variables (Pender, 1985; Stoner & Keampfer, 1985; Tilden & Weinert, 1987). Studies are based on different conceptual or theoretical bases and the literature remains largely unintegrated. The few chronic illness frameworks that have been developed did not evolve from studies of chronic illness but were adapted from other frameworks and applied to chronic illness (Craig & Edwards, 1983; Miller, 1983; Pollock, 1986).

What is needed is a theoretical framework grounded in studies of chronic illness that nurses can use to: (a) obtain insight and understanding into the problems particular to chronicity; (b) integrate and order much of the existing literature on chronic conditions; and (c) provide direction for building nursing models that guide practice, teaching, research, and policy making. The trajectory framework developed by Strauss and associates (Corbin & Strauss, 1988; Fagerhaugh & Strauss, 1977; Glaser & Strauss, 1968; Strauss, Fagerhaugh, Suzeck, & Wiener, 1985) is proposed as such a framework. It is based on years of studying the problems of chronic illness management both in the hospital and at home. It constitutes a substantive theory about chronic illness, developed specifically to provide insight and knowledge about chronic conditions in general. This research-based knowledge was never designed to be discipline bound; rather it was intended for use by any discipline in whatever manner might correspond to its purposes and functions. Over the years, many of this framework's concepts have been supported by research carried out by others (see, for example, Yarcheski, 1988). While the trajectory framework can potentially provide a means for integrating much of the nursing literature on chronic illness, the existing literature in turn can be used to densify and expand the theory. For example, research has been done examining the role that hardiness plays in adaptation to chronic illness (Kobasa, 1979; Pollock, 1986). Hardiness can be regarded as a condition that facilitates adaptation and therefore management, once the researcher understands the trajectory framework.

The purpose of this paper is to explain the framework and explore its usefulness to nursing. The first section of the paper is devoted to the framework itself. The second section examines its implications for nursing and offers the authors' conception of how these implications might be applied.

THE TRAJECTORY FRAMEWORK

The trajectory framework is a conceptual model built around the idea that chronic conditions have a course that varies and changes over time. This illness course can be shaped and managed. Shaping does not necessarily mean altering the direction of the course, though with some conditions this may be possible. Yet courses can be extended, kept stable, and their symptoms controlled through proper management. The shaping process is complicated, however, by the fact that much of the technology involved is extremely complex and has a potential for creating side effects. The illness and the technology used to manage it not only have consequences for the physical well-being of the afflicted individual, but also have consequences for biographical (identity over time) fulfillment and the performance of everyday life activities. In turn, consideration given to biographical needs and performance of every day life activities can affect the choices made about illness management and ultimately have consequences for the direction taken by the illness course. For example, a dialysis patient may find that adhering to a strict food and liquid intake is too difficult to follow; this will affect the treatment's effectiveness and ultimately the illness course. Or, a cancer patient may decide that the effects of treatment and their impact on quality of life are worse than the disease and refuse to undergo further treatment.

EVOLUTION OF THE FRAMEWORK

The trajectory framework has a long history going back some 30 years. It evolved both from a series of research projects about chronic conditions and from the practice of nurses, who brought to the classroom their experiences in the care of persons who had different chronic illnesses.

The application of the term "trajectory" to chronic illness came about because of an insight that Anselm Strauss, Barney Glaser, and a nurse, Jeanne Quint Benoleil, had while studying the care of dying patients. This was in 1960-1961 (Glaser & Strauss, 1965; Glaser & Strauss, 1968; Quint Benoliel, 1967; Strauss & Glaser, 1970). Their insight was that dying takes time, and that health professionals, families, and dying patients use many strategies to manage and shape the dying course. Looking for a way to conceptualize the phenomenon "management of an evolving course," the investigators decided to use the term "trajectory." In the spring of 1971, Strauss began to teach a course in Chronic Illness to graduate students. In this class, nurses were encouraged to present case studies of patients with chronic conditions for whom they had either given care or had interviewed. Also, doctoral students in both Nursing and Sociology were encouraged to undertake qualitative studies examining the management problems associated with different chronic conditions. These studies were published in a series of papers (Fagerhaugh, 1973; Reif, 1973; Wiener, 1975). They were later republished in a book by Strauss and Glaser (1975).

After several years, Strauss had accumulated a considerable body of knowledge regarding chronic illness. Looking for a way to pull it all together he began to formulate a theoretical explanatory framework, which then became the basis for his further teaching about chronic illness management. Nurses were then asked not only to present their cases in class but to analyze them, using this framework as a guide. At the end of each term, students were asked to interview someone with a chronic condition and to write a paper showing how they would use the framework to understand the management problems of the ill and to guide their own interventions.

Finding that the framework was helpful to those who used it, it was introduced in *Chronic Illness and the Quality of Life* (Strauss & Glaser, 1975). While the term "trajectory" was used to explain the illness course, however, trajectory as a framework was still rudimentary. There were few concepts, and their integration and development were minimal. In summary, the book pointed out that chronic conditions have a course that can be shaped through proper management. Also discussed was that chronic illnesses present certain everyday living problems (like managing regimens, reordering time, living with isolation, etc.) that must be managed if the ill and their families are to experience any sort of quality of life.

Then in the late 1960's, and in the 70's and 80's, Strauss and his associates (Corbin & Strauss, 1988; Fagerhaugh & Strauss, 1977; Strauss, Fagerhaugh, Suzeck, & Weiner, 1985) engaged in a series of studies regarding the management of chronic illness both in hospitals and at home. Since the focus of each study was different—pain, medical technology, and home care by couples—each study brought out different facets of chronic illness, their management and their implications, plus many details about the conditions that facilitated or hindered the management process. Each study validated previous findings and broadened the framework by adding new concepts and further developing and refining others.

For example, in the study of pain management (Fagerhaugh & Strauss, 1977) it was noted that persons admitted to the hospital with symptoms of pain are there because of some chronic condition. This means that the patients bring with them years of experience with pain management. Their experiences represent conditions that have the potential to affect pain management while they are in the hospital. Though staff may know a patient's medical history, they rarely have much knowledge about his or her experiences with illness, pain, or past treatments. Yet those experiences are very likely to influence patient-staff interactions and a patient's responses to care. Many patients are labelled as "difficult" because, unbeknownst to the staff, they are reacting in light of how their pain or other chronic conditions were handled in the past (Fagerhaugh & Strauss, 1977).

In a later study of technology, published as *The Social Organization of Medical Care* (Strauss, Fagerhaugh, Suzeck, & Wiener, 1985), it was found that chronic conditions frequently require complex technological intervention to prolong life and to shape the illness course. The use of this technology creates specialized problems of medical and nursing care. Patients also become more active participants, not only through the decisions they must make about treatment options, but also because they are called upon to remain still for long periods, engage in all sorts of preliminary preparations, and so forth (Strauss, Fagerhaugh, Suzeck, & Wiener, 1981, 1985). Also, machines and other forms of technology need to be tended to and monitored for safety (Strauss et al., 1985; Fagerhaugh, Strauss, Suzeck, & Wiener, 1987).

Since the use of technology tends to depersonalize care, there is an increased need to attend to the comfort of patients and their sentimental needs as well as those of concerned kin (Strauss et al., 1982, 1985). Then, too, someone must be responsible for coordinating the many types of care that a patient is receiving, like diagnostic tests and respiratory and physical therapy. The person responsible for this coordination is very likely to be a nurse.

Chronic Illness and the Quality of Life was revised (Strauss, et al., 1984), given the authors' now enlarged informational base about chronic illness. In this edition, the chronic illness framework was updated and expanded, the term "trajectory" becoming the central organizing concept of the book and its conceptual framework.

Turning to the management of care at home, the researchers brought out additional and very interesting features of managing chronic illness (Corbin & Strauss, 1988). Long narrative histories told by the ill and their spouses or domestic partners brought out several different trajectory phases (crisis, acute, stable, comeback, unstable, downward, and dying) through which chronic conditions may pass, as well as the differences in problems and management associated with each phase.

Furthermore, when one looks closely at how management is carried out over the years of an illness, it is clear that very little of it takes place in hospitals, rehabilitation centers, or other health facilities. Most of the day-to-day management takes place in the home and is carried out by the ill person and/or family. It is also in the home that the biographical consequences of illness and difficulties encountered in carrying out regimens (when these conflict with work or play) are most visible and talked about; also, the effort involved in making the necessary life adjustments becomes evident, such as when a cardiac patient must learn how to stay within the limits of a low sodium diet whether at home or while eating out (Corbin & Strauss, 1984, 1985a, 1985b). In the homes of the ill, we can also see clearly demonstrated the problems encountered daily as a result of the physical and mental limitations often accompanying chronic illness—for example, a sufferer from arthritis who struggles each morning to dress when joints are most stiff and painful (Corbin & Strauss, 1988, 1991).

After completing this later study, one of the authors (Corbin) was asked to teach a chronic illness course to R.N. students who had returned to study for their baccalaureate degrees. Most were working in hospitals and had come to the program with prior knowledge of the pathophysiology of illness. Corbin wanted to build upon that knowledge, and expand the students' knowledge of the problems associated with living with chronicity, as well as to raise their consciousness about the implications of that knowledge for the delivery of nursing care, whether that care takes place in the ICU or the home.

Corbin was at the same time making home visits to chronically ill clients in their homes. This was done through the Health Place, a nurse-managed center under the auspices of the Nursing Department at San Jose State University. Noting the complexity of the assigned cases, she looked for a way of conceptualizing the problems so that more comprehensive and effective care could be provided. Understandably she considered using the trajectory framework. While it had been applied to patients by nurses who had been students, and in papers that reflected their practice, no formalized systematic model of *nursing* care had ever been developed using the trajectory framework. For the framework truly to be useful for nursing practice, it would have to be converted from general chronic illness theory into a practical model that could be used by nurses.

VALIDITY AND WORTH OF THE FRAMEWORK

Before presenting the model that evolved, two questions will be addressed. First: Is the trajectory framework valid for understanding the problems associated with chronic illness and managing it? Second: Can this framework be used by nurses to develop models for care? In response to the first question, the authors believe it is a valid framework for chronic illness management. We say this for the following reasons: The framework is inductively derived, based on qualitative data that have been obtained from (a) a variety of sources, (b) multiple numbers of patients with different chronic conditions, and (c) collected in a variety of settings over many years. The sources include studies by Strauss and associates, as well as data provided by nursing students.

The research method used for building the theory was "grounded theory" (Glaser, 1978; Glaser & Strauss, 1967; Strauss, 1987; Strauss & Corbin, 1990). This particular method was actually developed during and as a result of the Glaser and Strauss research on dying. The method uses qualitative data obtained through observations, records, and interviews, case presentations, documents, biographies, and other sources, to generate concepts and their definitions, and to uncover relationships among the concepts. The procedures of grounded theory are designed to discover phenomena and their properties, uncover the conditions that bear upon those phenomena, explore the actions that are taken to manage, and elicit the range of possible consequences that may occur when action is taken or fails to occur. Theory builders are also directed to determine what happens to phenomena and related action when conditions change.

A strong feature of the grounded theory method is that hypotheses regarding the relationships between concepts are generated and provisionally tested against data *during* the theory development process itself. These hypotheses must hold up to scrutiny in case after case. When a negative case is found, then it is necessary to explain the conditions leading to this variation.

This research method also has specific procedures for both data collection and for analyses, which, if followed, meet the criteria for doing "good" science (Corbin & Strauss, 1990b; for more details about the procedures see Glaser, 1978; Glaser & Strauss 1967; Strauss, 1987; Strauss & Corbin, 1990).

The second question is: Can it be used by nurses? This concerns the practical worth of the framework.

CRITERIA FOR JUDGING THE PRACTICAL VALUE
OF A THEORY

In their book on grounded theory, Glaser and Strauss (1967, pp. 237-250) identify four criteria that can be used for judging the practical worth of a theory. The first criterion is that the theory must closely *fit* the substantive area in which it will be used. Since this theory about chronic illness trajectories has come from studying chronic conditions—and many of its statements can be supported by the research of others working in the area of chronic illness—it can be said to meet this first criterion. The second is that the theory must be readily understandable. Since the books (especially the 1975 book) and papers in which the theory, all or in part, have been read and used by countless numbers of practitioners and even lay persons, it surely has some degree of understandability, as well as provides *insight* and *understanding* into the experience of chronic illness and its management. The third criterion is that a theory must be sufficiently general to apply to multiple and diverse situations within the substantive area. Since this theory about chronic illness derives from the study of many different types of chronic conditions, in different settings, and has been used with different types of foci, it surely is sufficiently general to be useful in application. A fourth is that it must give the user at least partial control over the structure and process of situations as they change over time. Since this particular theory specifies contexts, conditions, goals of action, and possible consequences, it gives users the means by which to predict and thereby control for desired outcomes. Naturally, because it is a general theory of chronic illness management and not specific to each and every disease process, the details as they apply to each specific case must be filled in by the persons who use it. The more these details can be worked out, the more effective will be the application of this theory and the more control for desired outcomes will increase.

This framework has had considerable practical application over the years by individual nurses and has been found to be effective in providing insight and guiding practice. [See also Lubkin (1986) and Jillings (1987), who have used it as a sensitizing framework.] Its systematic application in nursing practice, however, remains largely unexplored by appropriate research. Much work is still needed to develop it as a model for research, teaching, and practice. As Meleis (1985, p. 30) states: "The primary use of theory is to guide research. Through interaction with practice, guidelines for practice will evolve... Until empirical validation or modification is completed, theory could be given practical validation and could therefore be allowed to give direction to practice."

The only way that the trajectory framework can be validated as a model for nursing care is for it to be used by nurses in practice and research. Both will lead to further research questions whose answers can be used to add to or modify the theory itself, as well as determine its usefulness for nursing.

We are presenting the framework here for nurses to see, use, and evaluate. The guidelines for how it might be applied to nursing represent only the authors' point of view, of course. Others might use it differently, and quite possibly more creatively.

MAJOR CONCEPTS, DEFINITIONS, AND RELATIONSHIPS

Phenomena must be given conceptual names or labels in order to be useful. The choice of labels is often arbitrary. Some of the labels given to the minor concepts in this framework represent the actual words used by the ill and their kin when describing phenomena. Conceptual names obtained in this fashion are referred to by Glaser and Strauss (1967) as "in vivo codes." Other names were coined by the researchers, and these include the major concepts. Regardless of their origin, however, these labels are meant to stand for phenomena and are not specific to any particular discipline.

Major Concepts

The major unifying concept of this framework is "trajectory" which denotes an illness course. This concept unites all of the other conceptualizations in the framework. The others stand in relationship to it as dimensions of the illness course, conditions that bear upon its management, or as consequences of how that course is managed. The other major concepts are: trajectory phasing and subphasing; trajectory projection; trajectory scheme; conditions influencing management; trajectory management; biographical and every day living impact; and, reciprocal impact.

Definition of Concepts

Trajectory as the illness/chronic condition course requires the combined efforts of the affected individual, family, and health care practitioners in order to shape it. That is, to determine its eventual outcome, manage any symptoms, and handle associated disability. Trajectories are often uncertain. They can be graphed, but only in retrospect. For although each illness has a potential course, its details cannot be fully determined ahead of time. Much depends upon the individual, the action taken to shape that course, and the turn of events that occur.

Trajectory phasing represents the many different changes in status that a chronic condition can undergo over that course. For a listing and definition of each phase, see Table 1. Within each phase there are subphases. *Subphasing* indicates that not only is there the potential for daily fluctuations in the illness course, but also for the following to occur. While the overall phase might be upward (as in comeback), downward (as in deteriorating and dying), or even level (as in stable), nevertheless within any particular phase there might be periods of several weeks or even months that can be characterized as a reversal, plateau, upward movement or a drop.

Trajectory projection stands for a vision of the illness course. The meaning of illness, symptoms, biography, and time are all built in (Robinson, 1988). Persons wonder: What will happen, how long do I (she) have, how far will I (she) go, how long will it take, and what does this mean for me (her) and the kin? For example, for some persons receiving a diagnosis of cancer, this means death; thus they project a shortened and debilitating life course. This vision may motivate them to take immediate and drastic action. For others, the diagnosis might be a reason

TABLE 1. Definitions of Phases

Phase	Definition
1. Pretrajectory	Before the illness course begins, the preventive phase, no signs or symptoms present
2. Trajectory onset	Signs and symptoms are present, includes diagnostic period
3. Crisis	Life-threatening situation
4. Acute	Active illness or complications that require hospitalization for management
5. Stable	Illness course/symptoms controlled by regimen
6. Unstable	Illness course/symptoms not controlled by regimen but not requiring hospitalization
7. Downward	Progressive deterioration in physical/mental status characterized by increasing disability/symptoms
8. Dying	Immediate weeks, days, hours preceding death

for sitting back and letting the illness take its course. Each individual who comes into contact with the illness and its management—physician, nurse, affected individual, and family member—has his or her own trajectory projection and ideas about how it should be shaped, which is founded on knowledge, experience, hearsay, and belief (Thorne & Robinson, 1988).

Trajectory scheme refers to the plan designed to: (a) shape the overall illness course, (b) control any immediate symptoms, and (c) handle disability. The scheme includes not only the medical treatment plan, which often includes the use of very complicated forms of medical technology, but can also include alternative forms of treatment such as herbal therapy, acupuncture, unapproved drugs, controversial diets, prayer, meditation, positive thinking, and other strategies (Forsyth, Delaney, & Gresham, 1984).

Conditions Influencing Management

There are many conditions that affect how and to what degree someone's trajectory scheme is actually carried out (Kruse, 1987). The conditions vary in degree and type and can facilitate, hinder, or complicate the management. Among the most important of these conditions are the type, amount, and duration of the technology used and the number and type of side effects it produces.

Management can be greatly complicated by this technology. Other conditions that influence the management process are the presence or absence of *resources*, such as manpower, social support, knowledge and information, time, and money. Still other conditions include: past *experience* with a medical condition and its management; *motivation* to do what is necessary; *setting of care*, whether home or a health facility; *life-style* and beliefs; nature of the *interactions* and *relationships* between persons involved in trajectory managing, i.e., agreeable or showing conflict; *type* of illness or chronic condition and degree of *physiologic involvement*; and nature of the *symptoms* and the *political* and *economic climate* that affects health-related legislation.

Conditions range from the broadest, that is those that are most distant from an individual and family, to conditions that are closer to them and likely to directly impinge on their management of the illness. Political and economic climate are among the more distant categories. They affect legislation pertaining to health care and the public monies available for care. These apply to the public in general, whereas life-style and beliefs are examples of conditions that are closer in. They pertain to a particular set of individuals. Not every possible condition has been listed here. What is important to know is that there are many conditions that affect management, they are varied, and they come into play in different combinations and at different times to either facilitate or hinder the management process.

Trajectory management represents the process by which the illness course is shaped, through all its phases, by the trajectory scheme. This includes controlling symptoms and treatment side effects, handling crises, preventing complications, handling disability, and so forth (Schneider & Conrad, 1983). While the overall goal of management is maintaining quality of life throughout and within the shaping process, the actual scheme by which this is accomplished must be specific to the illness phasing.

In setting the goal, arrangements necessary to reach it must be considered. One must examine the nature of the tasks to be done, then make arrangements for the resources that will be needed, for who will carry out the tasks, in which setting, how, and what can be expected in terms of consequences. For example, the goal in making a comeback is to bring the ill person back to a productive and satisfying life within the boundaries of his or her limitations. This means that management tasks will not only be directed at physiologic stabilization and recovery, but also include rehabilitative ones termed "limitations stretching," and biographical ones called "reknitting" (Corbin & Strauss, 1991). Arrangements then are needed for carrying out all of those major tasks (Corbin & Strauss, 1990a), because without such arrangements there is the possibility that one aspect will be overlooked and eventually this will have a deleterious effect on completing the other two. With time, the arrangements for illness management usually become routinized. Persons have set times, places, and individuals designated for taking or assisting with the giving of medications, undergoing treatments, ways of handling diet and rest, and so forth.

The Biographical and Everyday Life Impact of Chronic Illness

Biography refers here to the life course, made up of the many aspects of the self. It is the temporal dimension of identity: Together the biography and the self constitute identity. *Biographical impact* refers to the manner in which these many aspects of self can be affected or altered by illness or its management, thereby changing the person's life course (Birrer, 1979; Bury, 1982; Charmaz, 1983; Maines, 1983). *Coming to terms* is the process of making the identity adaptations that are necessary in order to live with chronic conditions. It is viewed as a process, rather than an end state, because identity adjustments must be made over and over again in accordance with changes in the illness course.

Everyday life activities refer to the actions of daily living through which persons live out the many aspects of their selves. *Limitations management* is the term that denotes the alterations and adaptations by which persons carry out those activities (Locker, 1983; Zola, 1982). For an individual with arthritis, this may mean stretching, warming up the joints, and waiting for medications to take effect before dressing in the morning. For a person with cardiac disability, limitations management involves learning which activities are likely to bring on symptoms of angina, then making needed arrangements for modifying or avoiding such activity. Strategies include minimizing the climbing of stairs, avoiding a walk on cold windy days, and eating light meals when one has to go out afterwards. For a quadriplegic, managing limitations means arranging to have an attendant come each morning and at night to get him/her out of bed, dressed, prepared for the day, then get back into bed at night. It may be necessary to make arrangements with others in order to manage limitations, for instance, getting one's wife to prepare a light meal, or scheduling the time that an attendant comes in the morning and returns in the evening.

Reciprocal impact is a very important concept in the trajectory framework. It is the consequence component. Its purpose is to sensitize us to the complexity of management and the potential compounding of problems that can occur due to the interaction between illness, biography, and everyday activities.

Application of the Framework to Nursing

The trajectory framework offers nursing a foundation for developing a model of nursing care that is: (a) specifically geared toward the problems of the chronically ill, (b) comprehensive in scope, and (c) gives direction to practice, teaching, research, and policy. A model rests upon its philosophy, and the philosophic orientation to which the trajectory framework gives rise can be termed "chronicity." This term can most effectively be elaborated by discussing its implications for nursing's four domains of concern: the person, health, environment, and nursing.

The Person

From the youngest to the oldest, anyone can be afflicted with chronic conditions. Above all, persons want to prevent such conditions, or, if this is not possible, to keep them under control. Prevention and management require lifelong daily activities. Unless an individual is hospitalized, the everyday prevention and management activities rest with persons and their kin. Thus, persons and their families are active participants in the prevention and management processes, holding in fact primary responsibility for both.

Complicating the matter is the fact that prevention of illness and illness management take place within a context. This context includes not only the specific characteristics of an illness, its treatment, and an individual's response to both, but also the personal biographies and daily activities of persons. These activities often continue despite illness, or the potential for illness to occur, if life itself is to go on. A central feature of management consists of the choices made about how to live biographies and carry out the activities of daily living so that they might be compatible with the prevention and management of illness. When someone is actually chronically ill, the choices are more difficult, sometimes painfully so.

Health

The focus of care in chronicity is *not* on cure but first of all on the prevention of chronic conditions, then on finding ways to help the ill manage and live with their illnesses should these occur. Interventions are aimed at fostering the prevention of, living with, and shaping the course of chronic illnesses, especially those requiring technologically complex management, while promoting and maintaining quality of life. In order to maximize the effectiveness of interventions, these must take into account the interactive effects between illness, biography, and the performance of everyday life activities. Continuity of care is essential for long-term intervention effectiveness. Here "continuity" means more than just continued supportive assistance. It denotes thinking of illness as a trajectory, that is, of having a past and future, which must be given consideration when planning care in the present.

Environment

Since so many of the day-to-day activities of preventing and managing chronic conditions take place in the home, *this* should be conceived as the center of care (Strauss & Corbin, 1988). By contrast, the hospital, rehabilitation unit, and other health care facilities and services should be viewed as backup resources to be called upon to supplement and facilitate home care. Environments can change in tandem with changes in the illness phasing, some being more technologically oriented than others. It is important that an environment be made suitable for the person, as well as for the medical technology within it. Also the ill and their kin must be psychologically, intellectually, and technically prepared (how to use and maintain equipment) to make the transition between environments, such as from hospital to home or home to nursing home.

Nursing

The ultimate goal of nursing in chronicity is to help clients to shape the illness course while also maintaining quality of life. This dual goal can be achieved through the provision of a type of nursing care termed "supportive assistance." Nursing care is first directed at assisting with the prevention of illness and, should illness occur, with the proper management of the chronic condition, while giving consideration to biographical needs and the performance of everyday living activities. The targets of nursing care are the individual, family, community, and society. The nursing process provides the operational means for providing supportive assistance. Specific nursing actions include direct care and—just as important—teaching, counseling, making referrals, making arrangements, and monitoring. Since cure is not possible, the supportive assistance should be seen as an ongoing process that includes a "trajectory" orientation. It should shift in nature in accordance with the changes in clients' illnesses and families' living conditions, while always keeping in mind where clients have come from and where they might possibly go.

Nurses are adept at providing complex technical care. In the prevention and management of chronic conditions, however, they must be equally adept at teaching, counseling, monitoring, and arrangement making. Nurses have an opportunity to make a unique contribution when it comes to the care of the chronically ill. Of all the health professionals, only nurses have the skills, knowledge, and vision to organize and provide for the comprehensive and technologically complex care that chronically ill clients require.

SPECIFIC GUIDELINES

The concepts of the trajectory framework provide the concrete structure that gives direction to the nursing process. Complicating performance of the operations of the nursing process are the interactive effects of managing illness, biography, and daily activities as well as other conditions bearing on management that also tend to be multiple and interactive.

Usually there is not one single condition bearing upon that management problem, but the interrelationship among many conditions. Also since neither illness nor life is static, the nursing process must be flexible and responsive to change, and must provide alternative plans for handling contingencies. An example of such planning would be helping a diabetic person work out a means for managing a diet and medication schedule when away on business trips, or helping an elderly couple when the husband has Parkinson's disease to develop a list of kin and friends that they can rely on should the wife become temporarily ill.

The Process

Step 1: Locating the Client and Family and Setting Goals. Using the concepts as a guide, the first step is to locate both the client and family in relationship to the management process, i.e., is it adequate, effective, and comprehensive enough to meet the illness, biographical, and everyday life management needs of this case?

"Locating" by the nurse means identifying the management problem and giving a basis for establishing the specific goals of intervention. Due to the reciprocal nature of the relationship between illness, biography, and everyday life activities, the nurse should locate the client on all three of these dimensions—and look for any possible interactive effects among them.

Areas of location include: specific trajectory phasing and subphasing, past phases, and any symptoms and/or disability experienced within this phase; the trajectory projection held by each participant in the management process; the trajectory management scheme, including both the medical regimen and any alternative forms of care; how, where, to what degree, by whom, the scheme is being carried out and any consequences this may have; where each family member is involved in the "coming to terms" process; and, the arrangements that are in place for carrying out the activities of daily living.

Once locating is completed, the nurse is ready to establish the goals of management. Since the client and family are active participants in the management process, the setting of goals should be a mutual task, and the clients should be given sufficient information to make informed choices. Goals must be phase specific. They should be directed toward reaching desired outcomes for that phase, while keeping in mind quality of life as the most general goal.

Examples of goals that nurses might establish include:

1. To assist a client in overcoming a plateau during a comeback phase by increasing adherence to a rehabilitation regimen so that he or she might reach the highest level of functional ability possible within limits of the disability.
2. To assist a client in making the attitudinal and life-style changes that are needed to promote health and prevent disease.
3. To assist a client who is in a downward trajectory make the adjustments and readjustments in biography and everyday life activities that are necessary to adapt to increasing physical deterioration.
4. To assist the client who is in an unstable phase to gain greater control over symptoms that are interfering with his or her ability to carry out everyday activities.
5. To assist a client in maintaining illness stability by finding a way to blend illness management activities with biographical and everyday life activities.

Goals can be broken down into specific client-oriented objectives. Built into the objectives are the criteria that will be used to evaluate the effectiveness of each intervention. What is important here is to look at what takes places in the process (the steps) of working toward a goal, as well as the end to be reached, and to be realistic about what can be achieved in what time period, taking into consideration the desires, wants, and abilities of the client and family.

Step 2: Assessing Conditions Influencing Management. The next step is to assess the conditions that bear upon management of this case, i.e., to identify those conditions that facilitate management or those that are impeding the ability to reach management goals. This step is important because it provides the variables to be manipulated in the intervention process in order to reach goals determined earlier through the locating process.

Areas to be assessed include: the resources—time, money, energy, manpower, equipment, technology, knowledge, and so forth—that are in place or that are necessary to manage this particular case. Also important to assess are the setting of care, its appropriateness, as well as its capacity or lack of capacity to meet this client's and family's needs, given the specific phasing and subphasing of the trajectory. The nurse would want to know: The experiences that the client has had with the illness and its management, and how these might be affecting current management; the degree to which the client and family are motivated to carry out management at home and for how long; something about their life style(s) and associated beliefs; and, the nature of their interactions, especially in relationship to managing the illness. On a broader scale, it is important that nurses understand something about the larger economic and political issues that bear upon management, such as the legislation affecting hospital stay, supportive services available in a community, length of time that home care and services can be provided, and what is paid for or not, so that patients' questions can be answered accurately, and appropriate teaching and counseling are provided.

Step 3: Defining the Intervention Focus. The third step is to define the target of intervention, i.e., what conditions should be manipulated in order to assist the client to reach the desired goal. For example, if it is suspected that a client holds an inaccurate trajectory projection and accuracy is necessary for carrying out the medical regimen—a requisite for keeping the illness stable—then the nurse would want to assess the client's level of knowledge about the illness. How much knowledge does the client have, where did it come from, is it accurate, how does it fit in with what the client believes and values? If the projection was based on inaccurate knowledge or a misinterpretation based on values or beliefs, then the nurse could set about correcting the inaccuracies and exploring with the client the values and beliefs that lead to misinterpretation. The target of intervention should also be verified with the client and family, along with their suggestions for how the target might best be reached.

Step 4: Intervention. In this step, the nurse manipulates the condition in question, that is, alters it in some way through the provision of direct care, counseling, teaching, arrangement making, and so forth. If there is inaccurate information, the nurse could, through teaching, help the client achieve a more realistic trajectory projection. Moreover, since chronic conditions are incurable, changes in illness status and in biography and daily activities are inevitable. Therefore, it is important that the nurse realize when situations change and how these changes call for new approaches. Repeated, ongoing, and flexible types of intervention may be necessary to reach desired goals.

Step 5: Evaluating the Effectiveness of Intervention. Evaluation in "chronicity" is not a cut and dried or an easy process even when a nurse has clear goals and criteria for the management of a client's condition. The nurse is often trying to change life styles, or the ways that people carry out activities, or to find better ways of helping them carry out their regimens, or to make arrangements for services; so it can be very frustrating (for nurse and client alike) to expect immediate results through the interventions. It is more realistic and effective to look for progress toward change, rather than change itself—and sometimes that progress is very slow in coming and the signs of it are barely perceptible. A nurse working with the chronically ill has to learn to "plant seeds" and let them grow. The achievement of realistic goals often involves trying out many different types of interventions, waiting for the client to reach an appropriate state of readiness, and looking for the cumulative impact of interventions over time.

Also, interventions may not be long-lasting. Reaching a goal, such as "adjustment" or "coping" or even illness stability, lasts only as long as any of the major conditions remain the same. Changes in the illness, in biography, or the ability to perform activities of daily living can call for making new adjustments or having to cope all over again. Before labeling someone as "not coping," it is important to step back and determine whether the individual is indeed not coping, or if instead he/she is in a transitional period during which new conditions are being struggled with and emotionally and physically being worked out. Just as an intervention cannot be a one-time act, neither can evaluation be done just once. Clients and their families need ongoing monitoring of their management activities and supportive assistance whenever their efforts break down or when future planning becomes essential.

IMPLICATIONS

The model of chronicity based on the trajectory framework has implications for nursing practice, teaching, research, and policy making.

Practice

Since the majority of clients seen in hospitals, homes, and clinics today are suffering from some form of chronic illness, nurses need to develop a consciousness of what living with chronicity means to clients and to provide a mode of care that reflects that consciousness. The chronicity model based on the trajectory framework offers a philosophic orientation and a set of general guidelines for application to clinical situations. It remains for nurses working in different areas of nursing, such as cardiac care, kidney transplant, and cancer to work out the specific details of how the model can best be used in their practice. Only they can ultimately define how useful the model can actually be, as well as establish its limitations.

Research

Research will come out of practice. As nurses use the model in their own areas, questions will arise about chronic illness in general, the interrelationship between different variables (conditions) affecting management, and which interventions are likely to produce the most effective outcomes under which conditions. Through such research, the model will not only be tested but verified, modified, and densified in process.

Research can also be done to test the concepts of the trajectory framework itself and their relationships, with modifications made accordingly.

Teaching

It is through teaching that the philosophy of chronicity can be passed on to students, as well as those skills, e.g., counseling, teaching, arrangement making etc., that are so necessary for carrying out the mission of "supportive assistance." Whether nurses work in adult or neonatal ICUs, geriatric clinics, rehabilitation units or in homes, it is crucial that they carry with them the philosophy of chronicity and have the skills necessary to provide their clients with the type of care that chronicity implies.

This model can also help nurses to think in terms of nursing problems by focusing on what it means for patients to live with an illness and to manage it on a daily basis. A physician can warn a cardiac patient about angina and provide a prescription for an alleviating medication. A nurse can help a client to identify which activities of daily living are likely to bring on angina, work out ways to avoid or modify these particular activities, discuss the most efficacious use of medication to prevent and alleviate symptoms, and emphasize danger signals.

The trajectory model and each of its concepts provides guidelines for the organization of teaching about specific diseases as well as the problems associated with chronicity in general. For example, the concept of "trajectory" can be used to open a discussion about specific underlying causes and physiologic changes, the resulting symptoms and/or associated disability, and the usual course that an illness might take, all of which have implications for nursing care. Furthermore, the concept of "trajectory scheme" opens the way for discussion of the usual treatment procedures and the nursing management problems, such as side effects, that these can create.

Understanding something about the conditions that bear upon management can make nurses more sensitive about the conditions that are operating in a specific case, and by manipulating the specific conditions operating in this case can help nurses to tailor interventions to the client's problems.

Policy Making

The trajectory framework has far-reaching implications for policy decisions. Under the present health care delivery system, hospitals and nursing agencies are paid to have nurses perform technical tasks, whether that care is being delivered in the hospital or home. Less value is placed on the other vitally important nursing functions of teaching, counseling, working things out, arrangement making, advocating, meeting emotional needs, and so on, yet these are equally important when clients are ill with chronic conditions. The trajectory model directs attention to the crucial role of these nursing functions.

Indeed, the nursing care of those people requires a radical shift in philosophy, practice, teaching, research, and policy (Strauss & Corbin, 1988). Until such changes are made, patients with chronic conditions will continue to receive less than adequate care and will be more likely by far to have problematic illness courses. While changes in approach to the care of the chronically ill are occurring, they are slow and illness specific.

IN SUMMARY

The model of chronicity discussed in this paper is based upon the trajectory framework. It provides a philosophic orientation and a systematic approach for thinking about and intervening in cases of chronic illness. It provides a means for ordering the existing literature on chronic illness by fitting it under appropriate concepts. Finally, it gives direction for making changes in nursing practice, teaching, research, and policy.

REFERENCES

Birrer, C. (1979). *Multiple sclerosis: A personal view.* Springfield, Ill.: Thomas.

Bury, M. (1982). Chronic illness as biographic disruption. *Sociology of Health and Illness, 4*(2), 167–182.

Charmaz, K. (1983). Loss of self: A fundamental form of suffering in the chronically ill. *Sociology of Health and Illness, 5*(2), 168-195.

Corbin, J., & Strauss, A. (1984). Collaboration: Couples working together to manage chronic illness. *Image, 16,* 109–115.

Corbin, J., & Strauss, A. (1885a). Issues concerning regimen management in the home. *Ageing and Society, 5,* 249–265.

Corbin, J., & Strauss, A. (1985b). Managing chronic illness at home: Three lines of work. *Qualitative Sociology, Fall,* 224–247.

Corbin, J., & Strauss, A. (1988). *Unending work and care: managing chronic illness at home.* San Francisco: Jossey-Bass.

Corbin, J., & Strauss, A. (1990a). Making arrangements: The key to home care. In J. Gubrim & A. Sankar (Eds.) *The home care experience* (pp. 59–73). Newbury Park, CA: Sage.

Corbin, J., & Strauss, A. (1990b). Grounded theory research: Procedures, canons, and evaluative criteria. *Qualitative Sociology, 13*(1), 3–21.

Corbin J., & Strauss, A. (1991). Comeback: Overcoming Disability. In A. Albretch (Ed.) *Readings on Disability.* Greenwich, CT: JAI Press.

Craig, H. M., & Edwards, J. E. (1983). Adaptation in chronic illness: An eclectic model for nurses. *Journal of Advanced Nursing, 8,* 397–404.

Cronin, S. N. (1986). Health beliefs in compliant and noncompliant hypertensive clients. *Journal of Community Health Nursing,* 3(2), 87–97.

Dai, Y. T., & Catanzaro, M. (1987). Health beliefs and compliance with skin care regimen. *Rehabilitation Nursing, 12*(1), 13–16.

Dodd, M. J. (1984). Measuring informational intervention for chemotherapy knowledge and self-care behavior. *Research in Nursing and Health,* 7, 43–50.

Dunkel-Schetter, C. (1984). Social support in cancer: Findings based on patient interviews and their implications. *Journal of Social issues, 40,* 77–98.

Fagerhaugh, S. (1973). Getting around with emphysema. *American Journal of Nursing,* 73, 94–97.

Fagerhaugh, S., & Strauss, A. (1977). *The politics of rain management.* Menlo Park, CA: Addison-Wesley.

Fagerhaugh, S., Strauss, A., Suzeck, B., & Wiener, C. (1988). *The hazards in hospital care.* San Francisco: Jossey-Bass.

Forsyth, G.L., Delaney, K., & Gresham, M. (1984). Vying for a winning position: Management style of the chronically ill. *Research in Nursing and Health,* 7, 181–188.

Gillis, C.L. (1984). Reducing family stress during and after coronary artery bypass surgery. *Nursing Clinics of North America, 19,* 103–12.

Glaser, B., & Strauss, A. (1965). *Awareness of dying.* Chicago: Aldine.

Glaser, B., & Strauss, A. (1967). *The discovery of grounded theory.* Chicago: Aldine.

Glaser, B., & Strauss, A. (1968). *Time for dying.* Chicago: Aldine.

Glaser, B. (1978). *Theoretical sensitivity.* Mill Valley, CA: Sociology Press.

Jillings, C. (1987). Is chronic illness a relevant topic for the critical care nurse? *Critical Care Nurse,* 7, 14–17.

Kobasa, S.C. (1979). Stressful life events, personality, and health: An inquiry into hardiness. *Journal of Personality and Social Psychology, 37*(1), 1–11.

Kruse, A. (1987). Coping with chronic disease, dying and death—a contribution to competence in old age. *Comprehensive Gerontology, 1,* 1–11.

Locker, D. (1983). *Disability and disadvantage: The consequences of chronic illness.* London: Tavistock.

Lovejoy, N. (1986). Family responses to cancer hospitalization. *Oncology Nursing Forum, 13,* 33–37.

Lubkin, I. (1986). *Chronic illness: Interventions for health professionals.* Boston: Jones and Bartlett.

Maines, D. (1983). Time and biography in diabetic experience. *Mid-American Review of Sociology, 8,* 103–117.

Meleis, A. (1985) *Theoretical nursing Development Procedures.* Philadelphia: J. B. Lippincott.

Miller, J. F. (1983). *Coping with chronic illness: Overcoming powerlessness.* Philadelphia: F.A. Davis.

O'Connor, A. M. (1983). Factors related to the early phase of rehabilitation following aortocoronary bypass surgery. *Research in Nursing and Health,* 6, 107–116.

Pender, N. J. (1985). Effects of progressive muscle relaxation training on anxiety and health locus of control among hypertensive adults. *Research in Nursing and Health,* 8, 67-72.

Pollock, S. (1986). Human responses to chronic illness: Physiologic and psychosocial adaptation. *Nursing Research, 35*(2), 90–95.

Popkess-Vawter, S. (1983). The adult living with diabetes mellitus. *Nursing Clinics of North America, 18*, #4, 777–779.

Quint Benoliel, J. (1967). *The nurse and the dying patient.* New York: Macmillan.

Reif, L. (1973). Managing life with chronic disease. *American Journal of Nursing, 73*, 261–264.

Robinson, I. (1988). Managing symptoms in chronic disease: Some dimensions of patients' experience. *International Disability Studies, 10*(3), 112–119.

Schneider, J., & Conrad, P. (1983). *Having epilepsy: The experience and control of illness.* Philadelphia: Temple University Press.

Stoner, M. H., & Keampfer, S. H. (1985). Recalled life expectancy information, phase of illness and hope in cancer patients. *Research Nursing in Health, 8*, 269–274.

Strauss, A., & Glaser, B. (1970). *Anguish: The case history of a dying trajectory.* San Francisco: Sociology Press.

Strauss, A., & Glaser, B. (1975). *Chronic illness and the quality of life.* (1st ed.) St. Louis: Mosby.

Strauss, A., Fagerhaugh, S., Suzeck, B., & Wiener, C. (1981). Patients' work in the technologized hospital. *Nursing Outlook, 29*, 404–12.

Strauss, A., Fagerhaugh, S., Suzeck, B., & Wiener, C. (1982). Sentimental work in the technologized hospital. *Sociology of Health and Illness, 4*, 254–78.

Strauss, A., Corbin, J., Fagerhaugh, S., Glaser, B., Maines, D., Suzeck, B., & Wiener, C. (1984). *Chronic illness and the quality of life* (2nd ed.). St. Louis: Mosby.

Strauss, A., Fagerhaugh, S., Suzeck, B., & Wiener, C. (1985). *The social organization of medical work.* Chicago: University of Chicago.

Strauss, A. (1987). *Qualitative analysis for social scientists.* New York: Cambridge Press.

Strauss, A., & Corbin, J. (1988). *Shaping a new health care system.* San Francisco: Jossey-Bass.

Strauss, A., & Corbin, J. (1990). *Basics of qualitative method: Grounded theory procedures and techniques.* Beverly Hills, CA: Sage.

Thorne, S.E., & Robinson, C.A. (1988). Health care relationships: The chronic illness perspective. *Research in Nursing and Health, 11*, 293–300.

Tilden, V.P. & Weinert, C., (1987). Social support and the chronically ill individual. *Nursing Clinics of North America, 22*(3), 613–619.

Wiener, C. (1975). The burden of rheumatoid arthritis. *Social Science and Medicine, 9*, 97–104.

Yarcheski, A. (1988). Uncertainty in illness and the future. *Western Journal of Nursing Research, 10*(4), 401–413.

Zola, I. (1982). *Missing pieces: A chronicle of living with a disability.* Philadelphia: Temple University Press.

The Trajectory of Cancer Recovery

Diane Scott Dorsett, R.N., Ph.D., F.A.A.N.

Comprehensive Support Services for Persons with Cancer
San Francisco, CA

In response to the Corbin and Strauss illness trajectory framework, this paper offers a *recovery model* as a more relevant trajectory for cancer as a specific chronic disease and as a general framework for clinical science. As counterpoint, the course of recovery is considered as a separate but influential continuum vis-à-vis the course of illness. The text presents an overview of the nature and meaning of cancer as a chronic disease, an operational definition of the recovery model, and a comparison and contrast of the illness and recovery trajectory frameworks in terms of their philosophic nature, therapeutic approach and research and educational and health policy-making emphases with regard to the cancer experience. When fully grounded in recovery science, the recovery trajectory model is predicted to be the more therapeutically effective clinical approach for professionals who care for patients diagnosed with cancer and their families.

A trajectory is the curve that a body describes in space from origin to first point of impact. In this issue's focal paper, Corbin and Strauss have applied the trajectory concept to chronic illness, recognizing its course as one that varies and changes over time. Their model posits eight phases from crisis to dying in the illness 'curve,' with each phase reflecting reversals, plateaus, upward movements, and drops in illness parameters. In essence, the course of illness, according to their model, can be influenced by three factors: (a) *personal characteristics* such as self-identity, perception of the illness ("vision of the course"), ability and motivation to adjust, and limitations such as disabilities; (b) *influential conditions* or available resources, embedded in social attitudes and economic and political climates; and (c) *the management scheme* or the goals, plan, and intervention factors that shape the illness course. Moreover, Corbin and Strauss say that the illness course can be shaped through the knowledgeable and skillful management of both health care professionals and patients and their families as active participants. Since an illness provides structure and its trajectory defines its process, they recommend the trajectory framework of chronic illness as a useful model for nursing practice, teaching, research, and health policymaking.

The purpose of this paper is to suggest that the *course of recovery* is a more relevant trajectory for cancer as a specific chronic disease and as a general framework for clinical science. The application of recovery theory as the central focus in the clinical management of cancer patients suggests a subtle but major conceptual departure from the Corbin and Strauss model. As counterpoint, the course of recovery is viewed as a separate but influential force vis-à-vis the course of illness. The two frameworks will be compared and contrasted in terms of their philosophic nature, therapeutic approach and research, educational, and policy-making emphases with regard to the cancer experience. Overall, if illness is represented by the trajectory of a Scud missile, recovery is the Patriot.

Cancer, as a collective of over 100 diseases, is a chronic illness estimated to become the major cause of death in the United States by the year 2000. Traditionally, a cancer diagnosis has been regarded as a death sentence marked by pain and the loss of functional independence. With the advent of new chemotherapeutic agents and improved radiologic technology in the 1970s and the more recent wave of biologic response modifiers (BRMS) offering novel diagnostic and therapeutic possibilities for the future, cancer has been reconceptualized as a chronic disease characterized by episodic, acute morbidities. As such, the survival picture has changed, resulting in many more prolonged remissions and, in many cases, cure.

The point of origin of the cancer trajectory is, most commonly, at diagnosis. Indeed, cancer diagnosis presents a crisis, requiring a major shift in the individual's sense of self. Often, the diagnosed patient has come to the experience asymptomatic, with a view of himself as a healthy person who is able to cope effectively with routine daily life. Ironically, the physical distress associated with the illness is due, in large part initially, to treatment which begins abruptly, causing significant life interruption and disturbance. Cancer treatment is rigorous, demanding active participation in self-care and rapid adjustment to a new world, including its new language and a newly perceived trajectory of life span.

Overall, cancer is a family disease necessitating critical shifts in the system that are disorganizing and costly, both economically and interpersonally. The patient and his/her social support system begin the trajectory on the steep side of the learning curve with the goal of mastering the experience in the service of survival.

Recently published statistics from the National Cancer Institute (American Cancer Society, 1991) reveal that not all cancers end in the dying process. Early detection and improved treatment have resulted in an above-70%, five-year survival rate for those diagnosed with cancers of the thyroid gland, testis, uterus, urinary bladder, breast, prostate gland and for melanoma of the skin and Hodgkin's disease. These cancers represent approximately 40% of the over one million malignancies diagnosed annually in the U.S. Central to the understanding and interpretation of these statistics is that they describe the aggregate but are largely imperfect in the ability to predict the individual case. To wit, in a *New York Times* front-page story entitled "Changing View of Cancer: Something to Live With" (Lewin, 1991), a 78-year old cancer veteran of seven operations, 30 radiation treatments and 17 years of weekly chemotherapy is described as "...still going strong, enjoying life with her husband of 57 years, her children and her grandchildren." Another 17-year survivor said, "Medicine is geared toward trauma and cure, but if you're living with the results of cancer for 10 or 20 years, you need other kinds of help" (p. A8). She defines *stages of survival*, "...from the acute period at the beginning where you're rushing around and getting into treatment to the extended period when you may be finishing chemotherapy, to permanent survival when you are figuring out how you go on" (p. A8). These examples highlight a difference in perception from one that is illness-based, ending in death, to one that is recovery-based, oriented toward survival.

Traditionally, oncology clinicians have been disease-focused. Physicians are concerned with 'cell kill' and nurses have concentrated their efforts on assisting in medical treatment and, in more enlightened times, on treating the patient's illness. In this paradigm, the trajectory is cross-sectional rather than longitudinal, geared toward the short-term goals of patient compliance and disease remission. Rarely has the health care system continued to follow a patient for very long after treatment has been concluded. Either the patient goes into a remission of indefinite duration or continues with residual disease that either responds to palliative treatment or leads to end-stage disease and death. In all but palliative cases, the patient and family have been left to go it on their own until recurrence, when the treatment process begins anew. An example of a typical illness trajectory is that depicted by the course of Hodgkin's disease (Figure 1) (Baez, Dodd, & DiJuleo, 1991).

This traditional picture has been altered only recently by oncologists who follow patients by seeing them every three to six months for physical examination, blood profiles, x-ray and imaging scans and, in more recent times, marker tests. In this system, the individual is defined by the illness and how well the disease responds to treatment. It does not incorporate the recovery medium because it does not recognize its characteristics. The Corbin and Strauss model fits well with this orientation. It is based on the assumption culled from their 1975 book, "Chronic Illness and the Quality of Life," that chronic illness has a course that can be managed. Further, the illness trajectory can be subphased according to its progression over time into eight categories, each one having its own set of problems and issues for patients, families, and practitioners. Even the "stable" phase emphasizes that the illness course and its symptomatology are controlled by the "regimen." Overall, the illness trajectory has a downward slope when the illness becomes unstable, progressively deteriorates, and eventually ends in death. This model condenses the cancer experience into the time warp of symptom-driven illness remediated by medical treatment until death occurs.

In contrast, the recovery model invites the person into the framework as the focal emphasis. Again, there is a subtle but important difference in the two models. The Corbin-Strauss model emphasizes professional intervention as a potent shaper of the illness curve. The recovery model makes clear that the pattern of recovery informs any intervention schema and that the pattern of recovery must be described and understood first, before meaningful and effective intervention can be mobilized.

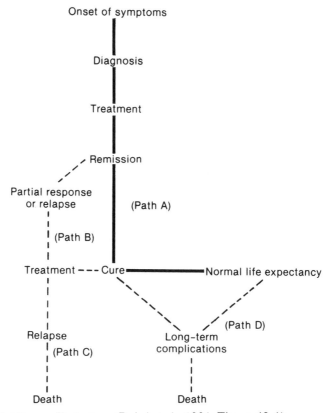

Figure 1. Disease Trajectory (Baird et al., 1991, Figure 43-1)

As with the illness framework, the recovery model has an operational definition: *Recovery* is a fundamental human process whereby change in well-being is
absorbed, assimilated, and accommodated over time in the service of both
survival and creativity. In the case of chronic illness, recovery begins at diagnosis
and continues until death, whether cancer related or not. The recovery process is
phasic, evidenced by a changing pattern of accommodations, attuned to a total
human response, including illness. Although the process of recovery may have
normative standards, each person's recovery is individual and uniquely defined.

Recovery is composed of three subprocesses that occur in simultaneity:
absorption, assimilation, and accommodation. *Absorption* involves the reception,
intake, and initial merger of information from both internal and external environments through all sensory media. Chemotherapy reception, including its half-life
phenomenon in the body, provides one example. *Assimilation* is the process by
which information is organized, incorporated, analyzed, synthesized, and assigned meaning. An illustration of this subphase is the patient's search for the
meaning of the cancer diagnosis in his/her life. *Accommodation* is characterized

by alterations, conformances, reconciliations, and, ultimately, major transformations representing the overall recovery emergence, such as with body image reintegration following cancer surgery.

The outcome of recovery at any moment in time is characterized by renewal and recuperation. In this sense, recovery incorporates the strength of the historical self and a new, evolving complexity in order to accomplish a major health transformation. Recovery has a continuum separate from but interactive with that of illness, whereby both illness and recovery courses are open and responsive to the influence of the other. Recovery is multidimensional, having physical, functional, cognitive, and affective dimensions that are interrelated by structure, process, and outcome manifestations.

Recovery can be assisted, facilitated, and strengthened through self-care and social, including professional, support. There is a broader and deeper opportunity for care-oriented practitioners to influence quality of life when recovery is the clinical focus. Understanding the process of recovery and how it influences the course of illness can more readily provide patients and their families with a greater sense of control. The framework for recovery is thus "user friendly," in that it enables an understanding that has an empowering effect. The recovery framework encourages collaboration and emphasizes cooperation rather than compliance. When complete with normative standards and related protocols, the recovery model is designed to be clinically useful due to both its specificity and multidimensionality. Thus, the recovery model represents an example of a framework broad enough to be heuristic, yet explicit enough to be practically effective.

The diagnosis of cancer represents the genesis of the recovery process, one that is phasic, beginning with diagnosis and continuing to the moment of death, whether it be cancer related or not. There is an important distinction between the illness and recovery frameworks here. The illness trajectory is described by a downward slope, with dying and death representing the last phase. In the trajectory describing recovery, the recovery process has its own phases, and continues up until the moment of death, signifying the remarkable human power to survive. The recovery model focuses on the recuperative powers of the individual when beset by illness. The model recognizes that the trajectory of an illness is governed in large measure by the therapeutic effects of the individual's recovery powers subsuming the patient's response to medical treatment. The recovery model emphasizes that although the illness has been a major factor in the individual's life transition, its chronicity or the nature of its longitudinal pattern over time is a function of recovery, not only the illness. It is in intervention strategies that guide the recovery process that therapeutic effect is most potently revealed. But before intervention can be designed, the normative process of recovery must be described.

For the care-oriented disciplines, as distinguished from those focused on cure, the Corbin-Strauss model suffers from the same imprecision as do other major theories that promise unification of the diverse conceptual universe created by chronic illness. The illness trajectory framework is as global as Fawcett's notion (1983) of nursing's four domains of concern: person, health, environment, and nursing. To wit, the authors defer to Fawcett's view when they discuss how the chronic illness framework applies to nursing. Given this crossover, Corbin and Strauss are proposing yet another global unification theory.

Recovery theory, on the other hand, may be thought of as a body of accumulating knowledge on a similar level of abstraction as is health promotion theory. The latter has as its central operative the duality of illness prevention-health promotion, whereas the recovery process shares in the same optimal wellness realm but operates more exclusively within recovery from illness parameters. Health promotion theory has achieved distinction due to its useful heuristic effect on clinical science. With maturation, recovery theory has the potential of leading to a similar result.

Currently, research into the recovery process is sparse and generally not grounded conceptually in a recovery framework as such. Its historical roots lie in cross-sectional, epidemiologic studies that offered information, revealing, for example, that approximately 20% to 30% of cancer patients will suffer emotional morbidity severe enough to require intervention six to eight weeks following diagnosis (Weisman, Worden, & Sobol, 1983). Another cadre of studies attempted to covary physiologic with psychosocial variables, as did Levy's work comparing blood levels of natural killer cells with scores on the fatigue and depression subscales of the Profile of Mood States inventory and with the patient's perception of her social support (1985, 1987, 1990). Intervention studies are even fewer in number, mostly anecdotal or, more recently, employing the case study or other qualitative methods.

To understand the recovery phenomenon and how clinical intervention may facilitate its progress, longitudinal studies of large cohorts utilizing a more common measurement base (both quantitative and qualitative) are required. Experimental protocols will need the normative base from the descriptive background generated in order to measure the effect of an intervention on the recovery process. Thus, to use the analogy once again, when the "curve" of the recovery (Patriot) trajectory is understood, the attempt to more effectively intercept the illness (Scud) trajectory will be more accurately and effectively executed. In this sense, intervention will be designed to strengthen the course of recovery and thereby 'shape' the trajectories of both illness and recovery, most potently revealed at their point of interception.

Published research into breast cancer, the most frequently occurring cancer in women and the most studied of all cancer categories, provides an illustration of how the recovery process may be documented. The results of five investigative teams working separately provide a beginning picture of how norms for cancer recovery may be established:

1. Scott and Eisendrath (1986, 1991) have described the early course of recovery in women with breast cancer over the initial 3-month period following diagnosis. Their study was designed to identify and document a pattern of recovery based on an empirical INTEGRATED CANCER RECOVERY MODEL (Figure 2), a matrix of four *interacting* dimensions of adaptation: (1) physical, (2) functional, (3) cognitive, and (4) affective. Findings indicated that in the 31 women studied, recovery improved across time in all state-type parameters, including physical symptom distress, functionality, and emotional distress. Trait-type characteristics such as self- concept and body image remained stable over the three-month period. Each evaluation time frame in this longitudinal study (in-hospital, and then, 10, 30, 60, and 90 days post-discharge) was found to be statistically different from all others, falling into the subphase categories of *acute* (in-hospital with highest distress levels); *relief* (steepest slope of improvement occurring over the first 10 days post-discharge); *stabilization* (during the first 30 days described by a recovery slope progressing at a slower rate); *quiescence* (lowest distress recorded in month 02); and, *pivotal or predictive* (implying a normalization evidenced by a trend toward either incline, decline or plateau during month 03). Moreover, throughout the three months, the women's sense of problem resolution remained uncertain, indefinite and doubtful, a decisively distressful element in their lives and in terms of the normalization trend.
2. Vinokur, Threatt, Vinokur-Kaplan, and Satariano (1990) studied 274 breast cancer patients longitudinally, evaluating the recovery process at 4 and 10 months following diagnosis. The study examined physical and mental

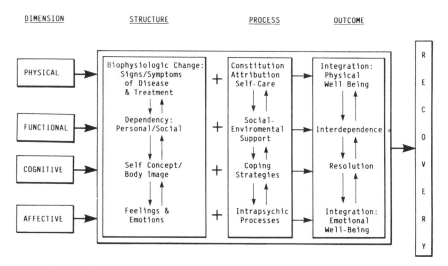

Figure 2. Integrated Cancer Recovery Model (Scott & Eisendrath, 1986)

health functioning, as well as factors predictive or facilitative of the recovery process. They found a significant, consistent improvement in the physical and functional aspects of recovery, but an arrest in the improvement in mental health and well-being indicators. Physical impairment at 4 months predicted the deterioration of mental health at 10 months, with women in the younger age group experiencing greater deterioration. Older women felt the impact of extensive surgery with more severe limitations in activity. In this study, the cognitive appraisal of threat was significantly predictive of psychosocial adjustment.

3. Dodd and associates (1991) conducted a study of the effect of self-care on symptom distress in breast cancer patients, most of whom were 14 to 24 months post-diagnosis. The women in this study were receiving chemotherapy for cancer recurrence. Over a three-month evaluation period from the start of their treatment, patients' emotional distress decreased despite a diminishing functional status and an increase in side effects of treatment.

4. A longitudinal study by Ell, Nishimoto, Morvay, Mantell, and Hamovitch (1989) examined psychological adaptation among 253 initially diagnosed breast, colorectal, and lung cancer patients at 3 to 6 months, 9 to 12 months and at a point 2 or more years post-diagnosis. They found that "...initial psychological status and other psychosocial factors and not illness-related factors, were predictive of subsequent adaptation." (p.406). Recovery was most arrested in those who remained distressed over time, as evidenced by declining mental health status.

5. Hislop, Waxler, Coldman, Elwood, and Kan (1987), in a prospective study of 133 diagnosed breast cancer patients, found that after four years, the levels of three variables, social interaction, anger, and cognitive difficulty, such as in concentration and making decisions, were not only significant prognostic factors for a host of psychosocial factors, but for both overall and disease-free survival as well.

Although these five investigative teams have conducted their work separately, the commonality of the constructs measured in all studies is quite evident: They are recovery, not illness oriented. Second, these projects utilize a longitudinal approach rather than the cross-sectional approach traditionally found in the literature. The linkage of these and other recent studies provides an example of how longitudinal research tracing the recovery process of cancer patients over time can provide a framework for understanding the recovery phenomenon, a foundation for building a predictive recovery model, and a heuristic base from which to tailor intervention strategies.

In order to shape national health care policy in an age of escalating cost and declining quality, a new and creative approach to the care of persons diagnosed with cancer and their families is demanded. As medical science develops more rigorous treatments to eradicate cancer, and administrators and third-party payers continue efforts to cut in-hospital stay time and to increase the ambulatory care of a sicker population, the concept of recovery becomes increasingly important. Complex cancer treatments, including bone marrow transplantation, will be provided in the near future on an outpatient basis. Attendant to this trend, the nonprofessional care partners of cancer patients will become responsible for their management in the home. The illness-medical treatment paradigm currently in place does not meet the emerging needs of this expanding group. The newly formed National Coalition of Cancer Survivors (NCCS) is making this increasingly clear as its members gather in greater numbers and in political strength.

Nurses, as healers, are in a prime position to take the lead in the effort to shape health policy. From a recovery rather than illness-oriented view, innovative health care services, grounded in the science of recovery, can be designed and established. As a consequence, expanded professional autonomy in nursing will result; for cancer patients and their families, services tailored to their central needs will afford continuous, high-quality care aimed at the promotion of more optimal health and quality of life, no matter its length.

In summary, a recovery trajectory framework has been proposed as a relevant model for cancer as a chronic illness. It has become clear from empirical evidence and from a growing body of literature that a science of recovery needs to be established. Educationally, courses in recovery, tailored to specific cancer populations such as cancers common in women, can be readily developed and based on information currently available. Recovery clinical services are desperately needed in this country for millions of cancer patients and their families.

As scientific research and educational practices begin to shape clinical services and interventions, national health policy will be challenged to develop a new blueprint for the health care system aimed at quality, affordability, accessibility and better use of resources. Although cancer as a chronic illness has provided the initiating critical event in this process, as in the economy, those factors that strengthen recovery will be key to the quality of healthy survival in the future.

REFERENCES

American Cancer Society (1991). Cancer Statistics, 1991. *Ca—A Cancer Journal for Clinicians, 40*(1), 3-32.

Baez, S. B., Dodd, M. J., & DiJuleo, J. E. (1991). Nursing management of persons treated for cure: Prototype—Hodgkin's disease. In Baird, S. B., McCorkle, R., & Grant, M. (Eds.), *Cancer nursing: A comprehensive textbook*, Philadelphia: W.B. Saunders Co., Chapter 43, pp. 673–688, Figure 43.1, p. 674.

Dodd, M. J. (1991). Personal communication. Unpublished data from the study "Self-Care and Side Effects of Cancer Chemotherapy," University of California, San Francisco.

Ell, K., Nishimoto, R., Morvay, T., Mantell, J., & Hamovitch, M. (1989). A longitudinal analysis of psychological adaptation among survivors of cancer. *Cancer, 63*, 406–413.

Fawcett, J. (1983). Theory: Basis for research and practice. *Proceedings of the American Cancer Society Third West Coast Cancer Nursing Research Conference, Portland, Oregon*.

Hislop, T. G., Waxler, N. E., Coldman, A. J., Elwood, J. M., & Kan, L. (1987). The prognostic significance of psychosocial factors in women with breast cancer. *Journal of Chronic Diseases, 40*(7), 729–735.

Levy, S., Heberman, R., Lippman, M., & d'Angelo, T. (1987). Correlation of stress factors with sustained depression of natural killer cell activity and predicted prognosis in patients with breast cancer. *Journal of Clinical Oncology, 5*, 348–353.

Levy, S., Haberman, R., Maluish, A., Schlien, B., & Lippman, M. (1985). Prognostic risk assessment in primary breast cancer by behavioral and immunological parameters. *Health Psychology, 4*, 99–113.

Levy, S., Herberman, R., Whiteside, T., Sanzo, K., Lee, J., & Kirkwood, J. (1990). Perceived social support and tumor estrogen/progesterone receptor status as predictors of natural killer cell activity in breast cancer patients. *Psychosomatic Medicine, 52*(1), 73–85.

Lewin, T. (February 4, 1991). Changing view of cancer: Something to live with. *The New York Times, 1*, A8.

Scott, D. W., & Eisendrath, S. J. (1986). Dynamics of the recovery process following diagnosis of breast cancer. *Journal of Psychosocial Oncology, 3*(4), 53–65.

Scott Dorsett, D., & Eisendrath, S. J. (1991). Early patterns of recovery in women diagnosed with breast cancer. Presented at the annual meeting of the Robert Wood Johnson Foundation-sponsored *Clinical Nurse Scholars Research Reports*, held at Camelback Inn, Scottsdale, Arizona, April 26, 1991.

Strauss, A., Fagerhaugh, S., Glaser, B., Maines, D., Suzeck, B., & Wiener, C. (1975, 1984). *Chronic illness and the quality of life*. St. Louis: Mosby.

Vinokur, A. D., Threatt, B. A., Vinokur-Kaplan, D., & Satariano, W. A. (1990). The process of recovery from breast cancer for younger and older patients. Changes during the first year. *Cancer, 65*, 1242–1254.

Weisman, A. D., Worden, J. W., & Sobel, H. J. (1983). *Psychosocial screening and intervention with cancer patients*. Boston: Harvard Medical School, Department of Psychiatry.

Using The Trajectory Framework: Reconceptualizing Cardiac Illness

Mary H. Hawthorne, Ph.D., R.N.

School of Nursing
Duke University

Cardiac disease is known to be the leading cause of premature morbidity and mortality in the United States. Nursing management of cardiac illnesses, as such, is a primary concern for most practicing nurses. Dramatic changes in cardiac patient populations and associated technology available for treatment indicate a need to reconceptualize the nature of cardiac illness and to consider alternative approaches to guide the care of these patients. Traditional care, to a large degree, has focused upon acute illness, consequently limiting needed attention to the increasing group of patients suffering chronic illness and disability.

In the present paper, the major changes in the cardiac patient population and in utilization of available technology are presented. The application of the Corbin and Strauss trajectory framework as an appropriate and useful framework for conceptualizing cardiac illness and care is then discussed. Five characteristics of the framework which render the model particularly well suited to address cardiac care are identified and discussed. These characteristics are: 1) comprehensiveness of care, 2) patient-centered care, 3) gender issues in care, 4) family-focused care, 5) technology and cardiac care.

Cardiac disease is known to be the leading cause of premature morbidity and mortality in the United States, with the majority of such illness being attributable to one disease entity, coronary artery disease (CAD). CAD, which alone accounts for an estimated 550,000 deaths and another 200,000 myocardial infarctions annually, is the leading cause of death and is responsible for more activity limitations than any other disease (American Heart Association, 1989; Eaker, Packard, & Wenger, 1986). The phenomenon of "heart attack," as such, probably remains foremost in the minds of most individuals when cardiac disease is contemplated.

Nursing care of patients with cardiac disease, however, encompasses a broad range of illnesses from very simple to complex, along with an array of associated symptomatology and suffering. Nurses may provide care for patients who are primarily asymptomatic and unlimited regarding desired life-style, for example, patients who present with essential hypertension. Assisting these patients to accomplish day-to-day living is not usually a concern; however, helping such individuals to achieve control of their hypertension, which constitutes a very real, yet insidious life threat, is a formidable challenge. Enabling these individuals to first appreciate the hidden risk associated with hypertension, and then to achieve necessary blood pressure control, requires individualized and creative nursing interventions (McEntee & Peddicord, 1987).

Nurses also provide care for many individuals on the opposite end of this continuum, i.e., those who are significantly ill and disabled. One such group are those patients, composed of people of all ages, who have reached end-stage cardiac illness due to a variety of diseases, such as coronary insufficiency, viral or idiopathic cardiomyopathy, valvular heart disease or congenital anomaly. These patients, who may be assisted at home with such complex interventions as intravenous administration of vasoactive agents (e.g., dobutamine), may struggle just to get through the day (Applefeld et al., 1983; Miller, Merkle, & Herrmann, 1990). As one of many important interventions, nurses may help these patients to remap activity patterns in order to conserve and ration very limited energy resources.

Taking center stage on this vast illness continuum has traditionally been the population of patients with acute cardiac illness secondary to CAD. The phenomenon of "heart attack," until recently commonly believed to be the leading cause of death and disability among males in their middle and most productive years, has been the focus of cardiac care in the second half of this century. An unprecedented effort has been mounted by the health care community in response to this health problem. Foremost among several successful treatment modalities are coronary artery revascularization (CABS), percutaneous balloon angioplasty (PCTA) and thrombolysis via tissue plasminogen activator (TPA). Many advances have also occurred in cardiac pharmacology, such as the development of calcium channel blocking agents that limit myocardial wall tension and oxygen consumption.

The end result of the utilization of such treatment options has been a steady increase in the number of patients surviving myocardial infarction. Thus, there has been a dramatic rise in the number of individuals surviving each year to experience end-stage disease and congestive heart failure (CHF) (Kaiser, 1986; Katz, 1987; Packer, 1987; Wilcox et al., 1988). In addition to pump failure, these patients often suffer from other disabling or life-threatening health problems, such as intractable dysrhythmias or renal failure. These conditions often require, in addition to frequent hospitalizations, complex and extended treatment.

The large concentration of resources which has been directed toward the treatment of acute coronary artery illness is a poignant example of the "cure"-oriented paradigm which has dominated health care in this century (Dubos, 1980). Although many of the benefits of "magic bullet" medicine are not inappropriate to or inconsistent with society's need to contend with a significant health problem, the application of such an approach has resulted in different, and perhaps more complex, clinical problems. These problems emerge as the unanticipated complement to the unprecedented success of such technology in prolonging survival. As more patients survive acute cardiac events, morbidity is compressed into the patient's future (Fries, 1986). When cardiac symptoms of disease recur, they are likely to be more complex, not only due to the side effects of the intervention employed for management of the acute illness, but also because the symptomatology is likely to be confounded by the effects of aging.

An important consequence of "cure"-oriented health care, then, has been to prolong the survival of cardiac patients through successful acute interventions, resulting in many older patients who experience more complex illnesses. At the same time, continued success and concomitant refinement of available technologies has enabled the extension of the use of such interventions to older and sicker patients. Older patients (over 65) presenting with congestive heart failure were once excluded from such invasive interventions as coronary revascularization. It is currently thought, however, that this subgroup of patients benefits significantly, not only in terms of symptomatic relief, but especially regarding the prolongation of life (Edmunds, Stephenson, Edie, & Ratcliffe, 1988; Gersh, Kronmal, & Schaff, 1985; Kaiser, 1986).

The evolution of increasing complexity in cardiac illness will most likely be significantly magnified by the evolving recognition by the health care community of the importance of CAD as the leading cause of death among women over 50 (Wenger, 1989). As an apparent gender bias is resolved, women are referred in greater numbers for invasive procedures (Eaker, Packard, & Thom, 1989; Gillum, 1987; Tobin et al, 1987; Wenger, 1990). These events are likely to occur later in the life span of women, as referrals for treatment have typically been initiated later in the individual's disease course. The patient's clinical response is therefore likely to be more complex, as it is confounded by the effects of aging (Kahn et al., 1990).

A synthesis of the available literature also suggests that the recovery trajectory for women following major cardiac events, myocardial infarction, and surgery, apart from obvious clinical differences and benefits, may be a significantly different experience from that of men (Boogaard, 1984; Gilliss, 1984; Murdaugh, 1986; Parchert & Creason, 1989; Penckofer & Holm, 1990; Wenger, 1990). Rankin (1989b), for instance, reported that women have significantly longer intensive care unit stays following coronary surgery than do men. Women also have been found to have a higher prevalence of incomplete revascularization, early and late graft occlusion, and recurrent angina (Becker, Corrao, & Alpert, 1988; Lazar, Wilcox, McCormick, & Roberts, 1987; Loop et al., 1983).

From the trends in patient populations and the application of technology for the treatment of cardiac illness, it seems reasonable to predict that the nurse will encounter increasing numbers of individuals experiencing extended periods of recovery, as well as disability, from cardiac illness. Future care of these patients will indeed address problems that cannot be obliterated through the application of technology alone. The traditional "cure"-oriented, acute illness paradigm is too narrow and shortsighted as an organizing framework for an increasing number of cardiac patients. A "cure"-oriented, acute illness paradigm is also inadequate in light of what has been learned about cardiac illness as a phenomenon. Traditional medicine has focused upon a disease model, which conceptualizes illness as a purely physiologic phenomenon. In contrast, however, illness has also been conceptualized as an experience that extends far beyond the presence of reducible physicochemical phenomena (Cassell, 1986; Good & Good, 1980; Kleinman, 1979). Perception of events, for example, has been found to significantly influence outcomes such as activity tolerance after infarction (Evart et al., 1986; Mishel, 1980; Peel, Semple, Wang, Lancaster, & Dall, 1962).

Given the trends in cardiac illness, along with what is known regarding the ineffectiveness of technology to "cure" coronary illness, caregivers are at a pivotal point where the needs and modes of care of cardiac patients must be revisited. A review of the Corbin and Strauss trajectory framework indicates that it is an appropriate framework with which cardiac care can be reconceptualized. A review of the model as applied to cardiac illness will be discussed in relationship to five key characteristics of the framework.

A CONTEXT FOR ILLNESS

Conceptualizing cardiac illness as a trajectory provides a comprehensive perspective which can have several advantages. By linking the person's past and projected future with the present illness, acute cardiac events are considered within a context. Frequently, acute cardiac events are thought of by the caregiver, as well as the patient, as discrete events lacking a tangible history (cause) or a future that may be altered or shaped (e.g., amenable to prevention).

This philosophical view is translated into care which is intervention focused and often fragmented. Patients, for example, are usually rotated around a hospital according to phase of illness and particular treatments needed. Patients may receive care from several different teams in several different care areas during a single hospitalization. This fragmentation and lack of continuity is a set-up for problems, as during each phase of the illness a new team must become familiar with the patient's complete history in order to deliver care based upon accurately interpreted data. Using Corbin and Strauss' trajectory framework in program planning for cardiac centers could stimulate the design of care delivery systems that minimize patient transfers within the hospital and identify consistent caregivers.

Thinking about cardiac illness comprehensively can also engender needed understanding of the potential illness course. As context enhances meaning, it underscores the importance of assisting the patient to plan for the future. Although the trajectory may be uncertain, it is possible to identify common, potential problems within certain patient groups around which rehabilitation programs can be constructed. This will become increasingly important as the numbers of patients experiencing end-stage cardiac disease increase. Accurately forecasting potential problems, such as volume overload in congestive heart failure, and teaching patients to self-manage intake and monitor body weight, has great potential for improving patient outcomes and reducing rehospitalizations.

Conceptualizing cardiac illness as a trajectory also emphasizes the importance of the role of cardiac-risk-factor modification in the prevention of disease (Cunningham, LaRosa, Hill, & Becker, 1990). This has significant implications, given the graying of America and the anticipated greater numbers of all individuals experiencing cardiac illness (Fries, 1986). This is particularly important in light of the evidence indicating that risk-factor modification can reduce mortality after myocardial infarction (Squires et al., 1990).

One of the problems that should be anticipated with the use of the trajectory framework is the possibility for dissonance between perspectives of the caregiver and the patient. As most individuals in American culture are likely to have been socialized in an acute illness paradigm, it may be difficult for the individual to conceptualize cardiac illness as a chronic disease trajectory. There is, for instance, evidence that some coronary surgical patients believe that the procedure may, indeed, effect a cure (Hawthorne, 1990). This is not difficult to appreciate in light of the fact that the procedure has been quite successful in eliminating for many patients their major symptom of illness, angina (Kaiser, 1986).

PATIENT-CENTERED CARE

An important advantage of the chronic trajectory framework is that because it is comprehensive, care must also be considered within the context of the patient's past experiences. This includes all past experiences, specifically the person's direct experience coping with cardiac illness. What this aspect of the framework accomplishes is to resolve the artificial dichotomy between the patient's time-line (biography) and the illness trajectory.

Care becomes, perhaps most important, person- rather than disease-focused when this dichotomy is resolved. This is very important in terms of nursing care, as patient needs can only be accurately identified from within the context of the individual and his/her interpretation of events (Paterson & Zderad, 1976). Interpretation of illness, as mentioned previously, is known to have a significant impact upon recovery outcomes from major cardiac events (Evart et al., 1986; Mishel, 1980; Peel et al., 1962).

A model of care that is patient-centered also places the control and accountability for shaping care and the illness trajectory into the patient's hands. This is important considering the increasingly chronic nature of cardiac illness, which may eventually shift the major focus of care away from the hospital and into the home. As this shift occurs, there will be a greater need for the patient to accomplish self-management tasks, incorporating the day-to-day contingencies and needs of family life. The concept of the patient not only being responsible for, but being able to shape the illness trajectory, is also a hopeful approach, as it supports the belief that the effects of illness and suffering can be attenuated.

Integrating biography with the chronic illness trajectory also allows the clinician to individualize care according to the patient's developmental needs. Understanding the individual's developmental needs is helpful in discerning the meaning of illness and in gaining insight into the person's priority setting and decision-making. Understanding the interaction between illness and developmental trajectories will continue to be a challenge as the population of cardiac patients becomes both older and more complex.

CARDIAC ILLNESS AND GENDER

The changing gender composition of the coronary-artery disease population raises important issues regarding developmental needs of cardiac patients. The "typical" coronary patient has been male, experiencing his first symptoms of illness during the middle years (Eaker et al., 1989). The male patient often suffers his first major cardiac event during his most productive years, when he is likely to be at a developmental crossroads (Tamir, 1983). A major cardiac event can in many aspects simulate a mid-life crisis, including such activities as value reorientation and "taking stock" of oneself (Hawthorne, 1990).

Statistics indicate, however, that women usually experience cardiac illness later in their life course than men (Eaker et al., 1989). The presentation of illness in women is reported to be more subtle, exhibiting first as angina, whereas a male is more likely to present initially with infarction. Since disease occurs later in life in women, it is quite possible that the meaning of the illness may differ according to age expectations, as Neugarten (1979), for example, posits that illness is perceived as an expected, hence normal event in the older patient. Research concerning the responses of women coronary artery surgery patients supports this view, as these patients report less mood disturbance and life disruption from illness than their male counterparts (Hawthorne, work in progress; Rankin, 1990).

There are also role issues related to gender and the cardiac patient that deserve serious consideration. The available research indicates that the recovery trajectory for women following major cardiac illnesses may be a different experience for them than for men. Boogaard (1984), for example, found that women and men resume different types of activities in different phases of recovery after myocardial infarction; men allow themselves a period of "passivity" or no activity, whereas women begin nonaerobic household activities soon after hospital discharge.

This information suggests that women and men utilize different cues and parameters to guide activity resumption. The multiple roles that women assume and the needs of others can significantly influence self-care and the resumption of activity. There is also added stress during recovery due to these demands (Rankin, 1989a). These data are consistent with what is currently understood regarding gender and role differences in response to illness (Baker, 1989; Hibbard & Pope, 1983; Verbrugge, 1979).

Women may also have special needs in managing chronic illness within present society related to family structure and demographics. Older women are more likely to outlive their spouses; these women frequently live alone and have limited resources for caregiving. Male patients, typically younger, usually have their spouses available to care for them during a major illness (Rankin, 1989a).

FAMILY-FOCUSED CARE

Enabling care to be structured from the patient's perspective also considers the importance of family in cardiac illness. Major cardiac events are known to generate much stress and are a significant disorganizing force within the family. These effects, for example, are thought to last for approximately six months after coronary revascularization (Gilliss, 1984). Attending to the needs of the family is important, as the patient's satisfactory psychological adjustment to major cardiac illness has been linked with family function, specifically to marital satisfaction (Dracup, 1985). Patient compliance with risk factor modification prescriptions has also been linked to spouse anxiety, as well as to level of marital functioning (Miller, Wikoff, McMahon, Garrett, & Ringel, 1990).

The family will assume greater importance as the population of cardiac patients becomes older and more complex. Caregiving responsibilities for elder and disabled individuals become more difficult as partners become ill or are no longer available to provide support. As noted earlier, widowed cardiac patients may suffer from lack of emotional as well as tangible supports, such as an available caregiver. Adult children of disabled patients, even when willing, may be unable to provide needed care, as most families now require dual incomes.

THE TRAJECTORY AND TECHNOLOGY

One of the appealing and useful aspects of the trajectory framework is that it allows for the dynamic and, more often than not, uncertain nature of cardiac illness. This is particularly true of current cardiac care, due in large part to the significant impact of available treatment upon the patient's illness trajectory. For example, the patient recovering from revascularization reaches a completely novel phase on his illness trajectory, where major symptoms of illness may be obliterated. Conceptualizing a realistic trajectory projection, replete with the demands that may be placed upon the patient during recovery, cannot be easily visualized under such conditions. A major role for nursing with these patients is to help make trajectory projections less abstract, thus making the self-management role tangible for the patient (Dracup, 1985; Hawthorne, 1990).

Expanding treatment options in cardiac care are also responsible for generating a more elaborate decision tree for the management of cardiac illness, replete with the opportunity for more phases and subphases and concomitant uncertainty. With thrombolytic therapy available almost universally, a "heart attack" or coronary thrombosis does not always mean an infarction; patients may literally avert or delay an infarction. Patients with significant (life-threatening) coronary occlusions may also avoid surgical intervention through the use of coronary angioplasty.

The down side of the use of these interventions is that data are still pending concerning long-term results. This is especially true regarding the effectiveness of coronary angioplasty. Thus, patients may experience significant uncertainty and anxiety regarding what their future will hold. Feelings of uncertainty can also be aggravated by the emergent nature of cardiac illness. These factors need to be considered, along with the significant emotional overlay due to the symbolic meaning assigned by western cultures to the heart as the major organ of life and the seat of all emotions.

One of the difficulties that technology and cardiac care present for the trajectory model, although the center of care ultimately is the patient's home, is that it is logical to predict that a major element of cardiac care will consist of the use of complex technology, at least for the foreseeable future. The use of such technology does affect the perspective of the caregiver, so that it is difficult to remain focused upon the home as the major site of the patient's care. This is true for the nurse in the acute care facility who must provide care that is exceedingly technological while helping the patient remap self-management strategies. This planning must often take place within a significantly abbreviated time frame (hospital course).

Another twist to the effects of technology upon the trajectory framework is the subpopulation of critical illness, the "chronically critically ill," which has ironically begun to emerge over the last decade. These patients are a group who have prolonged intensive care unit stays because of complications or underlying chronic illnesses (Daly, Rudy, Thompson, & Happ, 1991). Patients can spend literally months in highly cost-consumptive intensive care units. Despite their heavy dependence upon specialized care and mechanical support, recovery is often a reasonable hope for many. Not surprisingly, these patients are older, and likely to be in the end-stage disease subgroup. It appears that the fruits of modern medicine are such that most medical centers will be challenged with the care of such patients for at least the foreseeable future. It would be interesting to apply the trajectory framework as a model for the care of this emerging patient population.

CONCLUSION

The Corbin and Strauss chronic illness trajectory framework has been considered, within the confines of this article, as a model for care of cardiac patients. The examination of the trends in cardiovascular care indicates that the very successes of technology demand a broader framework to address patient needs. A framework is needed that places the patient at the center as the ultimate "shaper" of his trajectory, with illness considered within the context of biography.

The most apparent difficulty, however, with the use of the trajectory framework for cardiac care is the very technological nature and hospital base of the major treatment modalities. The use of such apparently powerful technology reinforces the medical paradigm of acute illness. As such, the treatment of major cardiac illness overshadows the fact that these acute episodes, albeit important influences upon the illness trajectory, represent only a small fraction of the time and effort patients expend managing a major illness. Nurses, who are uniquely qualified to understand this phenomenon, are in the position to assert the needed leadership to refocus care goals and the allocation of scarce resources. The trajectory framework demonstrates much promise as a needed model for achieving this objective.

REFERENCES

American Heart Association (1989). *1989 Heart Facts*. Dallas, Texas: American Heart Association.

Applefeld, M. M., Newman, K. A., Grove, W. R., Sutton, F. J., Roffman, D. S., Reed, W. P., & Linberg, S. E. (1983). Intermittent, continuous dobutamine infusion in the management of congestive heart failure. *American Journal of Cardiology, 51*, 455-458.

Baker, C. A. (1989). Recovery: A phenomenon extending beyond discharge. *Scholarly Inquiry for Nursing Practice, 3*, 181-194.

Becker, R. C., Corrao, J. M., & Alpert, J. S. (1988). The decision to perform coronary bypass surgery in women. What are the facts? *American Heart Journal, 116*, 891-893.

Boogaard, M. A. K. (1984). Rehabilitation of the female patient after myocardial infarction. *NCNA, 19*, 433-440.

Cassell, E. J. (1986). The return to ideals. *Daedelus, 115*, 185-208.

Cunningham, S., LaRosa, J. H., Hill, M. N., & Becker, D. M. (1990). The epidemiological basis for risk factor reduction. *Cardiovascular Nursing, 24*, 33-35.

Daly, B. J., Rudy, E. B., Thompson, K. S., & Happ, M. B. (1991). Development of a special care unit for chronically critically ill patients. *Heart & Lung, 20*, 45-52.

Dracup, K. (1985). A controlled trial of couples' group counseling in cardiac rehabilitation. *Journal of Cardiopulmonary Rehabilitation, 5*, 436-442.

Dubos, R. (1980). *Man adapting*. New Haven: Yale University Press (Original publication 1965).

Eaker, E. D., Packard, B., & Wenger, N. K. (1986). Coronary heart disease in women: A summary of the proceedings. *NHLBI Administrative Report* (pp. 1-45).

Eaker, E. D., Packard, B., & Thom, T. J. (1989). Epidemiology and risk factors for coronary heart disease in women. In P. S. Douglas (Ed.), *Heart disease in women* (pp. 129-145). Philadelphia: F. A. Davis.

Edmunds, H. L., Stephenson, L. W., Edie, R. N., & Ratcliffe, M. B. (1988). Open-heart surgery in octogenarians. *New England Journal of Medicine, 319*, 131-135.

Evart, C. K., Stewart, K. J., Gillian, R. E., Kelemen, M. H., Valenti, S. A., Manley, J. D., & Kelemen, M. D. (1986). Usefulness of self-efficacy in predicting over-exertion during programmed exercise in coronary artery disease. *American Journal of Cardiology, 57*, 557-561.

Fries, J. F. (1986). The future of disease and treatment. *Journal of Professional Nursing, 2*, 10-19.

Gersh, B. J., Kronmal, R. A., & Schaff, H. V. (1985). Comparison of coronary bypass surgery and medical therapy in patients 65 years of age or older. *New England Journal of Medicine, 313*, 217-224.

Gilliss, C. L. (1984). Reducing family stress after coronary artery bypass surgery. *NCNA, 19*, 103-113.

Gillum, R. F. (1987). Coronary artery bypass surgery and coronary angiography in the United States, 1979-1983. *American Heart Journal, 113*, 1255-1260.

Good, B. J., & Good, M.-J. D. (1980). The meaning of symptoms: A cultural hermeneutic model for clinical practice. In L. Eisenberg & A. Kleinman (Eds.), *The relevance of social science for medicine* (pp. 165-169). Boston: D. Reidel Publishing Co.

Hawthorne, M. H. (1990). An interpretive study of the metaphors male coronary artery surgery patients use to describe the surgical experience. (Doctoral Dissertation, Adelphi University, Garden City, New York, 1989.) *University Microfilms International.*

Hawthorne, M. H. (work in progress). *Coronary artery bypass surgery in women.* (Research funded by the School of Nursing, Duke University.)

Hibbard, J. H., & Pope, C. R. (1983). Gender roles, illness orientation and use of medical services. *Social Science and Medicine, 17*, 129-137.

Kahn, S. S., Nessim, S., Gray, R., Czer, L. S., Chaux, A., & Matloff, J. (1990). Increased mortality of women in coronary artery bypass surgery: Evidence for referral bias. *Annals of Internal Medicine, 112*, 561-567.

Kaiser, G. C. (1986). Lessons from the randomized trials. *Annals of Thoracic Surgery, 42*, 3-8.

Katz, N. (1987). Expectations of coronary artery surgery. *American Family Practitioner, 35*, 181-194.

Kleinman, A. (1979). Medicine's symbolic reality. *Inquiry, 16*, 203-213.

Lazar, H. L., Wilcox, K., McCormick, & Roberts, A. J. (1987). Determinants of discharge following coronary artery surgery. *Chest, 92*, 800-803.

Loop, F. D., Golding, L. R., MacMillan, J. P., Cosgrove, D. M., Lytle, B. W., & Sheldon, W. C. (1983). Coronary artery surgery in women compared with men: Analyses of risks and long-term results. *Journal of the American College of Cardiology, 1*(2), 383-390.

McEntee, M. A., & Peddicord, K. (1987). Coping with hypertension. *Nursing Clinics of North America, 22*(3), 83-592.

Miller, L. W., Merkle, E. J., & Herrmann, V. (1990). Outpatient dobutamine for end-stage congestive heart failure. *Critical Care Medicine, 18*(1), 530-533.

Miller, P., Wikoff, R., McMahon, M., Garrett, M. J., & Ringel, K. (1990). Marital functioning after cardiac surgery. *Heart & Lung, 19*, 55-61.

Mishel, M. (1980). Perceived ambiguity of events associated with the experience of illness and hospitalization: Development and testing of a measurement tool. (Doctoral Dissertation, Claremont Graduate School, 1980.) *University Microfilms International.*

Murdaugh, C. (1986). Coronary heart disease in women. *Progress in Cardiovascular Nursing, 1*, 3-8.

Neugarten, B. L. (1979). Time, age and the life cycle. *American Journal of Psychiatry, 136*, 887-894.

Packer, M. (1987). Prolonging life in patients with congestive heart failure: The next frontier. *Circulation, 75* (Suppl. IV), 1.

Parchert, M. A., & Creason, N. (1989). The role of nursing in the rehabilitation of women with cardiac disease. *Journal of Cardiovascular Nursing, 3*, 57-64.

Paterson, J., & Zderad, L. (1976). *Humanistic nursing*. New York: John Wiley & Sons.

Peel, A., Semple, T., Wang, I., Lancaster, W. M., & Dall, J. L. G. (1962). A coronary prognostic index for grading the severity of infarction. *British Heart Journal, 24*, 745-760.

Penckofer, S. M., & Holm, K. (1990). Women undergoing coronary artery bypass surgery: Physiological and psychological perspectives. *Cardiovascular Nursing, 26*, 13-18.

Rankin, S. H. (1990). Differences in recovery after cardiac surgery: A profile of male and female patients. *Heart & Lung, 19*, 481-485.

Rankin, S. H. (1989a). Women as patients and caregivers: Difficulties recovering from cardiac surgery. *Communicating Nursing Research, 22*, 9-15.

Rankin, S. (1989b). Women recovering from cardiac surgery. *Circulation, 80*, 211-391.

Squires, R. W., Gau, G. T., Miller, T. D., Allison, T. G., & Lavie, C. J. (1990). Cardiovascular rehabilitation: Status 1990. *Mayo Clinic Proceedings, 65*, 731-755.

Tamir, L. M. (1983). *Men in their forties*. New York: Springer Publishing Co.

Tobin, J. N., Wasserthiel-Smoller, S., Wexler, J. P., Steingart, R. M., Budner, N., Lense, L., & Wachspress, J. (1987). Sex bias in considering coronary bypass surgery. *Annals of Internal Medicine, 107*, 19-25.

Wenger, N. K. (1989). Coronary heart disease in women: Clinical syndromes, prognosis, and diagnostic testing. In P. S. Douglas (Ed.), *Heart disease in women* (pp. 173-186). Philadelphia: F. A. Davis.

Wenger, N. K. (1990). Gender, coronary artery disease and coronary bypass surgery. *Annals of Internal Medicine, 112*, 557-558.

Verbrugge, L. M. (1979). Female illness rates and illness behavior: Testing hypotheses about sex differences in health. *Women and Health, 4*, 61-79.

Wilcox, R. G., Von Der Lippe, G., Olsson, C. G., Jensen, G., Skene, A. M., & Hampton, J. R. (1988). Trial of tissue plasminogen activator for mortality reduction in acute myocardial infarction: Anglo-Scandinavian study of early thrombolysis (ASSET). *Lancet, 2*, 525-530.

Applying the Chronic Illness Trajectory Model to HIV/AIDS

Kathleen M. Nokes, Ph.D., R.N.

Hunter College, CUNY
Hunter-Bellevue School of Nursing

The Corbin and Strauss chronic illness trajectory model is particularly helpful in explaining the different phases of HIV (Human Immunodeficiency Virus) disease, since this infectious process is characterized by both phases and subphases. The model is not particularly helpful in identifying when the illness trajectory begins, since the model starts with the onset of symptoms, and HIV disease is characterized by a long, symptomless phase. The importance of politics and economics is also underestimated when applying this model to HIV disease. While this model presupposes the existence of support systems as being significant others, HIV disease is unique in that whole family systems may be eliminated by this infectious process, i.e., the typical pattern of HIV disease in the 1990s is that of a father dying from AIDS, a mother sick with HIV disease, one or more siblings infected, and one or more siblings coping with tremendous losses at a very young age.

AIDS/HIV, while continuing its course among gay/bisexual men and drug-using populations, is increasingly affecting women and children, racial and ethnic minority populations, heterosexuals, and people living in smaller cities and rural areas (CDC, 1991). HIV (Human Immunodeficiency Virus) disease is an infectious process which continues to impact on the host over many years. There is no cure once the person is infected with HIV, and the ability of medications such as zidovudine (AZT) to prolong survival is uncertain. The trajectory framework was developed to give direction for practice, teaching, and research in the area of chronic illness. A chronic illness model is currently applicable in examining this infectious disease. Should vaccines be developed which prevent the spread of HIV, this picture will change.

The Corbin and Strauss trajectory framework is built around the concept that chronic conditions have a course that varies and changes over time. Three stages of HIV infection have been identified. These are: the early or acute phase, which lasts weeks; the middle or chronic phase, which lasts years and is characterized by minimal but measurable pathologic changes; and, the final or crisis phase, which lasts months to years depending, at least in part, upon the efficacy and availability of treatment (Baltimore & Feinberg, 1989). HIV continues to replicate at a variable rate within the host from the time of infection until death.

An illness trajectory may be said to begin with the onset of symptoms (Corbin & Strauss, 1988). HIV disease begins long before the onset of symptoms. While some persons experience flu-like symptoms during the six-week period after infection, many do not know that a specific behavior such as unprotected sex or sharing of drug use equipment resulted in HIV-infection. It is only after many years that symptoms appear which hint at the underlying immune deficiencies. Unless clients seek out HIV antibody testing, they have no reason to suspect that they are infected. It is estimated that only 10% of the approximately one million HIV infected Americans know that they are infected. The initial symptoms which are sometimes referred to as ARC (or AIDS-Related Complex) are also vague if viewed in isolation. When a clinician takes a full history, the suspicion of HIV infection may emerge. Many people, however, especially women, are unaware that their sexual partner placed them at risk of HIV infection and so deny risk behaviors. The onset of symptoms cannot, therefore, be used to determine the onset of the illness trajectory for persons with HIV disease.

Trajectory phasing refers to the changes in status that a chronic condition undergoes throughout its course. The overall phase of HIV disease is downward, but the slope is barely perceptible for long periods of time. From the onset of HIV infection to the development of symptoms, the host's immune response is gradually impaired, but there are few, if any, objective symptoms of this deterioration. Both the characteristics of the host and virulence of the strain of HIV are believed to impact on the course of illness. CD4 blood cell testing and anergy panel testing are used to determine the phase of HIV disease. Clients with significantly depressed CD4 lymphocytes are believed to have been infected with HIV for a number of years. CD4 blood cell levels determine whether drug treatments such as zidovudine and aerosol pentamidine should be initiated. Anergy panels, consisting of PPD and at least two controls, determine if the client is capable of generating an immune response. Clients who are anergic are thought to be significantly immune depressed. The end-stage of HIV disease, namely Acquired Immune Deficiency Syndrome (AIDS), is associated with very low CD4 blood cell counts which result in severe depression of the immune response.

The trajectory model suggests that there are subphases within each phase that reflect daily fluctuations. A person's immune system adapts to challenges by hundreds of different antigens every day. When HIV impairs the immune response, these daily stresses can result in the development of symptoms. If the underlying damage to the infected person's immune system is not considerable, these symptoms may resolve spontaneously or with supportive treatment. This fine balance between symptoms and apparent health can be illustrated by examining lymphadenopathy in HIV infected persons. Cervical lymph nodes often enlarge when clients complain of upper respiratory infections or inhale drugs such as crack or heroin. When the cold is resolved or the drug use stopped, the cervical lymph nodes regress in size as long as the client's immune system remains somewhat intact. If the immune destruction is massive, then the cervical lymph node enlargement may be permanent. Subphases within phases may also extend for periods of several weeks or even months. The subphases of HIV disease from onset of infection until death range over even longer time periods. The first phase of HIV infection usually extends over a six-week to six-month period from infection to the development of antibodies against HIV. During this phase, some persons may experience subphases characterized by short periods of acute, flu-like illness. The second phase is thought to last several years and may be characterized by brief subphases of vague symptoms which are later associated with HIV infection. During the last phase of HIV disease, AIDS, there are subphases where clients who have experienced opportunistic infections, such as pneumocystis carinii pneumonia (PCP), can return to work and resume productive lives.

The trajectory projection stands for a vision of the illness course and reflects the meaning of illness, symptoms, biography, and time for each person affected by the illness. The trajectory projection in HIV disease has two distinct components. Initially the vision addresses the issues involved in first learning that one is HIV positive, and then the vision changes when one finally develops AIDS. After the initial devastation at learning that one is HIV positive, clients often feel hopeful about maintaining their immune system and avoiding AIDS. They speak of long-term survivors of HIV disease who are still healthy, and make changes in their lives which promote healthier life styles. Health care providers promote this hopeful attitude by stressing the importance of good nutrition, educating about HIV disease in order to empower clients to feel greater control over their infection, and advocating medications that slow down the infection of new CD4 cells. The vision changes when the client achieves an AIDS diagnosis according to the Centers for Disease Control criteria. There is a subtle shift as clients and health care providers admit that the immune system destruction is vast, and hopefulness is tempered by a different reality.

The trajectory scheme refers to the plan designed to shape the overall illness course, control immediate symptoms, and handle disability. The scheme includes both medical and alternative treatments. Eight years of the HIV epidemic passed before any medical treatments were approved for HIV disease. Even now, medical treatments of HIV disease are extremely limited, both by their effectiveness and also by difficulties in gaining access. Many HIV-positive clients use a variety of approaches, especially when trying to decrease symptoms of HIV disease such as skin rash or thrush. Alternative therapies are widely used by HIV-positive clients (Irish, 1989). Since there is no cure for HIV disease and limited accessibility to treatment, infected persons will try whatever seems to work. At this point in the HIV epidemic, there is no overall plan. The trajectory scheme for the HIV-infected person within the United States is chaotic, uncertain, and often characterized by mistrust of the medical research establishment.

According to the Corbin and Strauss article, one of the most important conditions influencing management of the trajectory scheme is the type, amount, and duration of the technology used and the number and type of side effects it produces. While this is a significant condition influencing management, it is certainly not among the most important for the HIV illness trajectory. A year's treatment with zidovudine costs approximately \$3,000 to \$8,000; aerosol pentamidine to prevent pneumocystis carinii pneumonia can cost \$600 per monthly treatment. Those who have the economic resources can access the technology.

Corbin and Strauss say that politics and economic climate are among the more distant categories affecting how the management of the trajectory scheme is implemented. For HIV-infected persons, these categories are the most significant. Use of specific treatments depends more upon geographic area, knowledge and attitude of the health care provider, economic resources, and social support network than on the effectiveness of the treatment. One client, who was a former IV drug user, asked this writer if she would have access to the cure when it was found or "would we be forgotten out here in Brooklyn." Although the cumulative incidence per 100,000 of diagnosed AIDS cases in the population within the United States is second highest in Puerto Rico (Washington, DC, has the highest cumulative incidence per 100,000), zidovudine is not accessible in Puerto Rico to those whose health care costs are covered by Medicaid.

Corbin and Strauss identify other conditions affecting management of the trajectory scheme. These conditions include past experience with a medical condition; motivation; setting of care; life-style; and, degree of physiologic involvement. Each one of these conditions will be examined below from the perspective of HIV disease.

It is not unusual for clients with HIV disease to have members of their extended family and friends diagnosed with HIV disease and perhaps to have died from AIDS. Newly diagnosed persons with HIV often know more about the course of the illness and its treatment than some health care providers. The client may have been the primary caregiver for a sexual partner who recently died from AIDS or may have shared drug use equipment with a close group of four to five friends, all of whom are now dying or have died from AIDS. A client may have buried a husband from AIDS, be caring for a two-year-old child with HIV disease, and coping with the symptoms of HIV disease herself. Because of the client's prior experiences with HIV disease, the health care provider cannot shield him or her from the knowledge of an uncertain future. The client is sometimes fatalistic about the course of HIV infection and the effectiveness of available treatments, and this can cause discomfort for the health care provider.

Motivation is an important factor in managing the trajectory scheme for HIV disease. Some clients are motivated to stop drug use, to adopt healthy behaviors, and to feel optimistic about a cure. Others do not interface with health care providers and resume drug-using behaviors, sometimes to an even greater degree than before diagnosis. Some clients adopt safer sex practices, while others are angry that someone infected them and try to spread the virus to uninfected sexual partners. Safer sex and drug use practices are difficult to sustain, and relapses are common. The health care provider can assist clients to resume healthy behaviors and remotivate them by maintaining a caring attitude.

Setting of care is a significant condition affecting management of the trajectory scheme in HIV-infected persons. Home care is not a realistic option when the client lives on the street. Home care services cannot be placed in environments where clients continue to actively deal in illegal drugs and engage in violent behaviors. Compliance with the medical regimen can be difficult in a shelter situation where other clients steal medications in order to sell them. Gay male clients who have lived in urban settings and have enjoyed a long-term relationship may be forced to return to their childhood communities when the significant other dies. These gay clients may feel socially isolated and estranged from parents who are now opening their homes to them during the last days of their lives.

Degree of physiologic involvement is an important consideration in management of the trajectory scheme. Extreme shortness of breath associated with pneumocystis carinii pneumonia and weakness make maintenance of activities of daily living virtually impossible. The dementia associated with HIV can impair judgment. Decisions about health care, finances, and living arrangements may be increasingly inappropriate. While there is no concern with casual transmission of HIV, other organisms such as tuberculosis can be spread to others. A person may have more than one illness trajectory, with the second trajectory related or not related to the first (Corbin & Strauss, 1988). An HIV-infected client with AIDS may be managing illness trajectories associated with HIV-infection and two or three opportunistic infections along with cancer. An HIV infected client with AIDS may have pneumocystis carinii pneumonia, tuberculosis, herpes zoster, and non-Hodgkins lymphoma.

Trajectory management represents the process by which the illness course is shaped by the trajectory scheme. This includes handling disability. Women of child-bearing years who are diagnosed with HIV infection often have questions about how HIV will impact on their intense desire to bear children. The overall goal of trajectory management is maintaining quality of life by shaping the scheme specific to the illness phase. HIV-positive women with relatively intact immune systems seem to have successful pregnancy outcomes. If pregnancy is a desired goal in an HIV-positive woman, the scheme should be shaped so that the pregnancy occurs as early as possible during the HIV disease. The possibility of vertical transmission of HIV from the infected woman to the fetus also seems to be less during the early phase of HIV disease.

Reciprocal impact is an important concept in the trajectory framework, since it addresses consequences. Sharing information that one is HIV positive can have far-reaching consequences. Persons have been fired from their employment and therefore lost health insurance, income, and other benefits. The American Medical Association is currently advocating that HIV-infected physicians inform potential clients that they are infected. The consequences of sharing this information could be loss of patients, resulting in loss of income and ability to maintain a practice. In a climate of homophobia and racism, revealing information about HIV status can expose a person to overt and hidden discrimination.

The ultimate goal of nursing chronically ill persons is to help clients shape the illness course and maintain quality of life. In the first step, the nurse locates the client and family and sets goals. The nurse locates the specific HIV illness trajectory phase of the client by interpreting results of CD4 blood cell testing and the anergy panel. The nurse carefully elicits whether the client's history includes engaging in behaviors associated with HIV transmission and assesses for symptoms related to HIV disease. The nurse gives the client and significant others time to share their vision of the HIV trajectory course. The nurse collaborates with the physician and other members of the health care team and teaches the client and significant others about HIV disease and proposed treatment options. The nurse assesses conditions impacting on management of the client with HIV disease and makes referrals which ensure that the client receives necessary entitlements. Time is allotted for family members and significant others to share their concerns about casual transmission of HIV in the home setting. Ways to prevent spread through contact with infected blood are discussed explicitly. Goals are established which are phase specific and anticipate potential crises. Goals which will require a long period of time to achieve, such as establishing guardianship for a client's dependent children, are identified while the client is well enough to work on achieving them.

Step 2 involves assessing conditions influencing management of the client. This includes assessment of resources and setting of care. An HIV-positive client who is working will eventually be unable to work. This same, relatively well client who is living with her sister and three children in a one-bedroom apartment, may be unable to stay there when she becomes acutely ill. Because of the relatively long illness trajectory of HIV disease, the nurse needs to be aware of conditions affecting management of the client and to establish alternatives. Perhaps the client who can no longer work and needs assistance with activities of daily living can be maintained with her sister and the children if assistance is placed in the home. But perhaps the client's social support system will be overwhelmed and the client will live out her last days as a border in an acute care hospital. The nurse can attempt to manage the client's condition by identifying alternatives, but in some situations, options do not exist.

The third step is defining the intervention focus. Working with HIV-positive clients and their significant others can be overwhelming because the needs are so extensive. The nurse needs to be clear about the areas where nursing's contributions can make a difference and recognize that a very sad situation may persist despite the nurse's best efforts. One of the nurse's most important contributions to the care of the HIV-positive client and significant others is health teaching which focuses on clarifying misconceptions about transmission of HIV infection. The nurse's behavior toward the HIV-infected client can also serve as a role model for significant others who may be fearing to care for the client in their home. Nurses can empower HIV-positive clients and their significant others by teaching them about the management of their HIV illness trajectory and helping them to coordinate the maze of health care providers. Accessibility and continuity are two keys to quality management of the HIV illness trajectory.

The fifth step addresses evaluating the effectiveness of the intervention. The nurse working with HIV-positive clients needs to recognize that there are limits to strategies to change behaviors. When the chemically dependent client has a relapse or the sexually active client has unprotected sex, the nurse cannot evaluate the intervention as ineffective, but must recognize that a different approach is needed. Behaviors associated with staying healthy with HIV disease are difficult to maintain, and so relapse cannot be regarded as a failure but rather as a different subphase within that phase of the illness trajectory.

SUMMARY

Corbin and Strauss' illness trajectory model was applied to the nursing of clients with HIV disease. Essential concepts of the model were applied to the illness trajectory of HIV disease and, in some cases, the model did not describe HIV disease. For example, while Corbin and Strauss say that the onset of symptoms signals the beginning of the illness trajectory, this is not the case in HIV disease. Clients can be without any indication of infection for periods extending up to 15 years. The impact of politics and economics on the health care of HIV-infected persons is also underestimated. On the other hand, the concept of a trajectory projection and phasing is very helpful in understanding HIV disease. These clients often experience two visions — one when initially diagnosed as HIV-infected and the other when an AIDS diagnosis is received.

The Corbin and Strauss model was applied to nursing practice, teaching and research. The five steps of the nursing process were related to application of the illness trajectory model to caring for HIV-positive clients and their significant others. The Corbin and Strauss model has implications for teaching about HIV disease. The content in different courses could address nursing care of clients and affected others at different trajectory phases. For example, an approach consistent with trajectory phasing was used in developing the subspecialization in nursing of persons with HIV/AIDS within the graduate nursing program at Hunter College, Hunter-Bellevue School of Nursing. Nursing research can use this chronic illness model to develop new knowledge about effective strategies for HIV-infected clients and their significant others at different phases of the illness trajectory.

REFERENCES

Baltimore, D., & Feinberg, M. (1989). HIV revealed: Toward a natural history of the infection. *New England Journal of Medicine, 321,* 1673-1675.

Centers for Disease Control (1991, February). The HIV challenge continues. *CDC HIV/ AIDS Prevention.*

Corbin, J., & Strauss, A. (1988). *Unending work and care: Managing chronic illness at home.* San Francisco: Jossey-Bass.

Irish, A. (1989). Maintaining health in persons with HIV infection. *Seminars in Oncology Nursing 5,* 302-307

Chronic Mental Illness:
The Timeless Trajectory

Marilyn M. Rawnsley, D.N.Sc., R.N., C.S.

Teachers College, Columbia University, New York

Mental illness encompasses many dimensions. While the etiology of most major disorders remains unclear, their devastating effects are readily apparent. The substantive and practical value of the trajectory model of chronic illness is examined in relation to the characteristics of major mental disorders. Two clinical vignettes illustrating the timeless trajectory of chronic mental illness are analyzed with reference to the model's components. The potential utility of this model for revitalizing research and practice in psychiatric-mental health nursing is discussed.

Corbin and Strauss present a persuasive argument for the utility of a trajectory model for management of chronic illness. The description of the model's development is consistent with data grounded in the study of chronic illnesses whose symptoms primarily manifest as problems of physiological structure and function. While individual history and response complicate the professional challenge of shaping the illness trajectory, the fluctuating course within many chronic syndromes has been identified as having common phases or points of predictability.

But the category of chronic mental illness is inclusive of many disorders and dysfunctions whose etiology is unclear and whose disruptive patterns emerge as idiosyncratic puzzles. Can the trajectory model of chronic illness be applied to management of major mental illness without either stretching its credibility or oversimplifying the problems? The purpose of this paper is to address issues of validity and utility of Corbin and Strauss' trajectory model for explaining the illness course in persons who live with major mental disorders and to explore its implications as a guide for research, practice, and policy in the context of chronic mental illness.

BACKGROUND AND METHOD

Any investigative perspective incorporates strengths and limitations. It may be instructive, however, to report the methods by which the substantive and practical value of the trajectory model for nursing management in chronic mental illness were addressed. Two evaluative approaches were used. One strategy was to consider the logical consistency between the explicit and implicit assumptions of the model in relation to the characteristics of major mental disorders. Another was to investigate the goodness of fit between the components of the model and the lived experience of actual patients accomplished through a retrospective investigation of two clinical histories. The latter approach was aimed at testing the trajectory model on a "least likely to succeed" hypothesis. That is, if components of the model can be demonstrated to have relevance for major mental disorders with a guarded prognosis, then its potential as an organizing framework in less complex situations can be inferred.

In the psychiatric tradition, where participant observation (Gubrium, 1988) is a time-honored inquiry method, the experiential knowledge of the therapist is a primary data source. Truth value, or credibility, of the case material generated from this source is judged, as is all qualitative data, by its recognition as valid and meaningful by others who have had similar experiences (Guba & Lincoln, 1981).

The case study data used for analysis emerged from this respondent's 20 years of experience as a psychotherapist and clinical consultant in inpatient and outpatient psychiatric settings. From this professional knowledge base, two cases were selected that illustrate existential uniqueness yet provide a general representation of ways in which chronic mental illness can penetrate an unfolding biography and challenge the professional community. Although this respondent was professionally engaged with these patients at various points during their distress, their respective illness courses are a matter of interdisciplinary record. Pseudonyms are used to protect privacy, and some individual details are altered for confidentiality.

DECISION TRAIL

The general procedure for determining the validity and utility of the model in a mental health context was initiated by gaining a general understanding of the development and purpose of the chronic illness trajectory as described by Corbin and Strauss. In order to minimize the likelihood of a halo effect from an intellectual evaluation of the model on the perception of salient case material, narrations preceded further analyses. In other words, once the decision was made to respond to the model by constructing a type of ex post facto test of its utility for chronic mental illness, any interpretations of the relevance of the unifying concept of trajectory and its associated dimensions were postponed until case narrations were complete.

Following completion of the narrations, the degree of congruence between the model's premises and those that underlie current criteria for diagnosing major mental disorders in adults (American Psychiatric Association, 1987) was assessed for logical consistency. Then each case was examined for evidence of the postulated pattern of a chronic illness trajectory. Since each narration spans several years of clinical history, even a synopsis yielded many pages of transcription. In view of the space limitations of this paper, each case was edited into a clinical vignette after the complete narration was analyzed with reference to the components of the model. To ensure representativeness of the edited vignettes in preserving the integrity of the full narrations, a doctorally educated nurse unfamiliar with the trajectory model compared each vignette to its respective narrative for correspondence of salient features.

SUBSTANTIVE VALUE

The gaps in knowledge introduce opportunities for its advancement. If premises on which a theory or model is based cannot be demonstrated to be logically consistent with the phenomenon in question, however, then further analysis is irrelevant. Since the discussion of the model and the cited references indicate that it evolved out of studies of chronic illness with a physiological orientation (Corbin & Strauss, in this issue), a responsible stance in assessing its utility for mental illness is one of healthy skepticism. The issue is one of scope or generality; that is, can the conceptual parameters of the chronic illness trajectory model accommodate the phenomena intrinsic to major mental illnesses?

The idea that chronic conditions have a course that varies and changes over time is central to the trajectory framework. According to specified criteria of the revised third edition of *Diagnostic and Statistical Manual of Mental Disorders, DSM-III-R* (American Psychiatric Association, 1987), there are discrete diagnostic classifications that involve a manifestation of dysfunctional symptoms over a minimal duration of several months. These syndromes are ordinarily characterized by exacerbations and remissions. Symptoms and episodes in pretrajectory phase of major mental disorders, however, are frequently recognized as such only in retrospect; at the time they occur, they are often given a less pernicious diagnosis. Such initial judgments are not necessarily examples of professional ineptitude. Responsible clinicians are concerned about the social repercussion of labeling persons as suffering from major mental illness. Most important, errors on the side of caution are preferable to the alternative of instituting treatments to counteract effects of a major personality disorganization when less aggressive interventions would suffice.

Consequently, by the time symptoms have endured consistently enough for a major mental disorder to be confirmed, individuals may have progressed through several mini-trajectories, each of which was not actually a separate syndrome, but a disguised prelude. In summary, while this first assumption of the trajectory model is consistent with the standardized criteria for confirming mental disorder, explanatory knowledge of the phenomenology of mental illness does not provide sufficient information to avoid dilemmas of diagnosis.

The second premise is that the illness course can be shaped and managed, in the sense that it can be extended and kept stable through control of symptoms. This assertion is qualified by recognition of potential for medical technology to create undesirable sequelae that become a dimension of the management process. While there is indisputable evidence that medical therapies such as psychotropic drugs, electroconvulsive treatments, and the infrequently employed interventions of psychosurgery can induce problems of varying severity, it is less certain that the illness course in major disorders can be shaped to ensure the goal of maintaining quality of life. The conditions influencing management cited by Corbin and Strauss, that is, the resources of social support, manpower, knowledge and information, time, and money are of critical concern in chronic mental illness. Moreover, life-style, belief structures, and the capacity to engage in interpersonal relationships are likely to be severely compromised in major mental disorders, presenting per-plexing obstacles to forming a therapeutic alliance with professionals (Selzer & Carsky, 1990). Involving family members or significant others in limitations management in chronic mental illness requires a delicate balance of mutual needs in situations where personal relationships are already jeopardized (Atwood, 1990).

The third premise concerns what Corbin and Strauss term biographical fulfill-ment, or identity over time, and its impact on performance of activities of daily living. While a reciprocal effect between a chronic illness and the consequences of its treatment is acknowledged, this exchange seems predicated on a time-ordered connection that places onset of the disease before biographical impact. In mental illness, however, studies of early life conditions are finding empirical support for connections between childhood trauma and deprivation and adult psychiatric dysfunction (Gottshalk, 1990; Paley, 1988; Terr, 1991).

In mental disorders, identity over time may be the source of illness. In other words, sorting out the connections between mental illness and biography is somewhat of an etiological riddle (Gottshalk, 1990). While the effects of the disorder on the quality of life appear devastating to observers, symptom mani-festation can represent an attempt to resolve a long internal struggle to establish or maintain personal identity under overtly or covertly hostile environmental conditions (Paley, 1988; Terr, 1991; Thompson, 1990). Moreover, the perfor-mance of everyday life activities is central to evaluating the degree of dysfunction, efficacy of treatments, and meaning of biographical unfolding.

These selected issues clarify areas of congruence and areas of dissonance in characteristics of chronicity with a physiological origin as opposed to that with a psychogenic basis, but it seems reasonable to claim a partial degree of correspon-dence between the central premises of the trajectory model and salient characteristics of chronic mental disorders. Although there are dimensions which require further explication, the scope of the trajectory model is sufficiently general for application in the context of mental illness. Two clinical vignettes highlight its potential as a framework for guiding psychiatric-mental health nursing in chronic illness. (See Appendix.)

DISCUSSION

The events described in these cases, while manifesting characteristics unique to each client, are not unlike many accounts of chronic mental illness. More often than not, the course of major mental disorders is characterized by a capriciousness and confusion that invites, from the vantage point of dispassionate hindsight, many armchair opinions on how singular occurrences could have been better managed. The aim of this discussion, however, is not to second guess the facts. The point is to use these cases as common reference for addressing the question, "To what extent can the trajectory model of chronic illness be said to promote insight and understanding into the problems of chronicity as represented in these vignettes?"

Both stories illustrate conceptual compatibility between the general concept of trajectory and the lived experience of major mental disorder. In both situations, pretrajectory episodes escalated into acute psychotic states. The crises requiring hospitalizations are followed by periods of stabilization of varying duration. Ron's illness course more closely approximates the trajectory phases as described by Corbin and Strauss in the sense that a final deteriorating phase preceding his death is evident, although his death was not a direct result of schizophrenia, but of complications of a chronic physical condition precipitated by adverse response to neuroleptic medications.

Despite arbitrary conceptual boundaries of theory, a real human being lives as an integral whole. The reciprocal effects of mental disorder on physical well-being, particularly adherence to medical regimen, cannot be overemphasized. With notable exceptions, for example, suicide as a consequence of depression, ingestion of certain psychoactive substances or responses to auditory commands in psychosis, most persons suffering from mental illness die from other causes. Of course, early or untimely deaths may be associated with the presence of an underlying mental disorder such as inadvertent overdoses or fatal accidents that befall those who have difficulty in sorting out reality, death by exposure, and other misfortunes of homelessness. But statistics to support this hypothesis are unavailable or unreliable. What is known, however, is that some disorders with an onset in late adolescence or early adulthood are less apparent or at least, less obviously dysfunctional, in those who survive into older age (American Psychiatric Association, 1987).

While persons with chronic mental illness generally do not die of it, its magnitude is no less consuming. Rachael's situation is typical: exacerbations and remissions; difficulty distinguishing between the effects of the disorder and the effects of the interventions; temporary comebacks, but no restoration. These patterns are consistent with Corbin and Strauss' contention that a trajectory is uncertain and can be accurately graphed only in retrospect. Projecting a vision of the illness course in major mental disorders is complicated by the pervasive repatterning of personality.

The circular weave of psychosis diffuses direction. The capacity to make meaning out of current life events and incorporate them into a coherent biography is diminished when, in a desperate attempt to maintain an identity over time, current conditions are diffused into past pathology. When changes are unavoidable, they frequently precipitate a recurrence of acute symptoms. Chronic mental illness is an existential predicament, a way of being at odds in the world. Afflicted persons have described their life as "a living Hell." And just as in dramatic portrayals of that theological construct of eternal hopelessness, time seems suspended for those who struggle through decades with major mental illness. It is hardly hyperbole then, to characterize the chronicity of major mental disorders as a "timeless" trajectory, seemingly without purpose, without progress, without resolution and without end.

The erosion of resources, professional as well as personal, is more the rule than the exception. The affected individuals and their families, cited by Corbin and Strauss as holding primary responsibility for both prevention and management processes, have been only marginally functional before the illness became apparent. Like Ron, who eventually listed the "psychiatric staff" as his significant others, or Rachael, who maintains a delusional pursuit of her first counselor, mental illness at first distorts, and then destroys, the capacity for sustaining meaningful relationships central to identity over time. Locating the patient on the trajectory and setting attainable goals is a continuous challenge. The focus of intervention is always short term and realistic; it is aimed at keeping the individual functioning in activities of daily living with minimal distress to self and others. The longer the span between crises, the more successful the intervention.

Continuity of care, postulated in the trajectory model to be essential to long-term management effectiveness, rings of empty rhetoric in a mental health delivery system as impoverished and disorganized as its clients. The burden of providing predictable care for the majority of those severely disturbed citizens disenfranchised through their erratic way of being in the world falls on the public sector of health care. Mental illness has not lost its social stigma; public policy reflects that bias. Therefore, participation in the political process, to give voice to those who cannot speak out for themselves and to provide incentives for professionals to enter and remain in the field is central to the success of any framework for professional action in mental health. Public policy is the new frontier for progress in mental health.

There are important lessons to be learned from the past. The mental health reform efforts, spurred by the Federal Community Mental Health Act in 1963, resulting in de-institutionalization of the mentally ill, shifted the locus of responsibility for the chronically mentally ill from large dehumanizing central institutions to local agencies. The only real shift, however, was in statistics on the locus of the afflicted persons. With a reduction of more than 75% of state hospital beds for the mentally ill since 1955, it has been estimated that twice as many severely mentally disturbed people are on the streets as in the hospitals (Sage, 1990). Whether the motivation for this movement represents the heightened social conscience of the Sixties or whether it was an attempt at cost containment gilded in illusions of community is a matter of perspective and politics (Rawnsley, 1989). What is clear, however, is that a movement based on logistics rather than substantive knowledge has failed; yesterday's reform is today's disgrace.

Of course, the true test of utility is contingent upon outcomes from prospective studies that use the trajectory model to anticipate problems and evaluate intervention strategies for persons diagnosed as suffering from mental disorders with a long-term prognosis. Introducing the trajectory framework into the language of mental illness offers new directions for advancing knowledge in the field through action research.

Research-in-practice can elicit individual "pattern-specific" information recommended by Corbin and Strauss. Interpretations of findings from these clinical studies can suggest modifications for the trajectory scheme appropriate to nursing management of chronicity in mental illness.

The urgency to derive professional solutions, however, ought not eclipse the importance of theoretical development. Action research can proceed simultaneously with studies grounded in the phenomenology of chronic mental disorder. Studies designed to yield the same systematic observations that produced the model for chronic physical illness need to be conducted for mental disorders. Only through the richness of data generated from the realities of the lived experience of mental illness can the biases that now occlude professional vision be disclosed.

Bok (1990), commenting on the apparent discrepancy between the academic priorities of a discipline and its response to societal needs, identifies an inconsistency between social needs and social values. This divergence is manifested in the search for knowledge that is highly valued as judged by extramural funding, but not necessarily valuable in terms of social betterment. The impact of scientifically verifiable knowledge in shaping public estimation of a discipline's social image should not be underestimated (Bok, 1990). The trajectory model for chronic illness has interdisciplinary heuristic value as a tool of discovery and verification, e.g., generating new questions for study, demonstrating a difference in outcomes, and shaping a more positive public image of mental health as a humanistic science for social betterment.

IMPLICATIONS FOR PSYCHIATRIC-MENTAL HEALTH NURSING

One adventitious outcome of a bi-level approach to chronic mental illness through basic and applied research may be a revitalization of psychiatric-mental health nursing. The "revolving door" of repeated recurrence in mental illness can engender a sense of futility in professionals who work primarily with the chronically mentally ill. Attracting enthusiastic new graduates to a field permeated by cynicism is unlikely. Using the trajectory scheme to legitimize posing and solving new substantive puzzles may serve as an antidote to discouragement. Reframing the situation as a challenge to nursing scholars and practitioners to collaborate in discovery and action research introduces a balancing factor necessary to counteract the constriction to which all who work exclusively in psychotherapeutic modalities are susceptible (Greben, 1990).

Corbin and Strauss comment on the need for nurses to be as adept at counseling, teaching, monitoring and coordinating care as they are at providing complex technical care. What they term "supportive assistance" is the core activity of psychiatric-mental health nursing. As a specialty practice of the discipline, psychiatric-mental health nursing shares the professional value of contributing to social betterment through responsive rather than prescriptive service to clients. As a legitimate member of an interdisciplinary mental health team, nurses who work with the chronically mentally ill function not only as coordinators of client care, but also as primary therapeutic professionals. Now, as developments in neurosciences and biological psychiatry advance knowledge of physiological processes associated with mental disorder, different professional challenges are emerging (Gottshalk, 1990). Introduction of new medical technologies precipitated by these discoveries may accentuate, rather than diminish, the importance of a therapeutic alliance. The logical choice for this therapeutic responsibility is psychiatric-mental health nurses, not because they are the least expensive professional members of the mental health team, but because they are the best prepared to deal with the reciprocal impact of chronicity and its treatment in daily life. If the trajectory framework can facilitate the nursing management aspect of chronic mental illness, it will enhance the real work of psychiatric nursing, which is, and always will be, the therapeutic use of self.

CONCLUSION

While the theoretical struggles of psychiatric-mental health nursing aim at clarifying discipline-specific constructs, contemporary practice emphasizes a collaborative process. Ultimately, derivation of theoretical constructs for nursing research and practice in chronic mental illness consistent with Corbin and Strauss' trajectory model is embedded in its substantive web of significance for the interdisciplinary domain of mental health. But the preliminary interpretation disclosed through the retrospective analysis of actual cases indicates that the trajectory scheme for chronic illness postulated by Corbin and Strauss has practical value as an interdisciplinary grid for collaborative planning and monitoring of symptom control in mental illness, without eclipsing the theoretical pluralism inherent in the field.

Incorporating the trajectory model into the language of research, practice and education in psychiatric-mental health nursing could signal an exciting 'comeback' of professional and public interest in promoting quality of life for those who are living the timeless trajectory called chronic mental illness. Moreover, it could lead to a restoration of respect for those professionals who are committed to caring for persons whose struggle to make meaning out of life seems to estrange them from everyone, including themselves.

REFERENCES

American Psychiatric Association. (1987). *Diagnostic and statistical manual of mental disorders, DSM-III-R*, (3rd ed., revised). Washington, DC: Author.

Atwood, N. (1990). Integrating individual and family treatment for outpatients vulnerable to psychosis. *American Journal of Psychotherapy, 40*(2), 247–255.

Bok, D. (1990). *Universities and the future of America*. Durham, NC: Duke University Press.

Corbin, J. M. & Strauss, A. (1991). A nursing model for chronic illness management based upon the trajectory framework. *Scholarly Inquiry for Nursing Practice, 5,* 9-28.

Gottshalk, L. (1990). The psychotherapies in the context of new developments in the neurosciences and biological psychiatry. *American Journal of Psychotherapy, 40*(3), 321–339.

Greben, S. (1990). The importance of balance in the practice of psychotherapy. *American Journal of Psychotherapy, 40*(1), 37–43.

Guba, E., & Lincoln, Y. (1981). *Effective evaluation*. San Francisco: Jossey Bass.

Gubrium, J. (1988). *Analyzing field reality*. Beverly Hills, CA: Sage Publications.

Paley, A. M. (1988). Growing up in chaos: The dissociative response. *American Journal of Psychoanalysis, 48*(1), 72–83.

Rawnsley, M. (1989). Learning to grow through loss: A focus for preventive mental health services. In S. Klagsbrun, G. Kliman, E. Clark, A. Kutscher, R. DeBellis, & C. Lambert (Eds.), *Preventive Psychiatry* (pp. 11-16). Philadelphia: Charles Press.

Sage, D. (Producer). (1990, October 30th). Broken minds (Frontline, Documentary). New York, NY: Channel 13.

Selzer, M., & Carsky, M. (1990). Treatment alliance and the chronic schizophrenic. *American Journal of Psychotherapy, 40*(4), 506–515.

Terr, L. (1991). Childhood traumas: An outline and overview. *American Journal of Psychiatry, 148*(1), 10–20.

Thompson, T. (1990). The evolution of schizoid orality. *American Journal of Psychoanalysis, 50*(3), 1990.

APPENDIX

CLINICAL VIGNETTES

Vignette #1 — Ron

Ron's first acute episode occurred in his senior year of college. A few months before, he had seen a psychiatrist for an intermittent distress diagnosed as occasional panic attacks accompanied by mild agoraphobia (American Psychiatric Association, 1987). As he began the drive home after classes, unexpected snow squalls hit the area, reducing visibility to less than a few yards. By mistake, Ron turned north on the highway rather than south, heading toward the mountains and into the snow belt. As the geographical boundaries faded, and ego boundaries loosened, Ron concluded that his psychiatrist had arranged this experience to help him deal with his fears. Several hours later, he was found wandering about a ski resort town, disheveled, disoriented and actively hallucinating. His parents, both of whom were in their early sixties, arrived at the psychiatric unit of the community hospital within a few hours after Ron's admission. They were attributing his "nervous breakdown," to studying too hard and worrying about getting a good job when he graduated. Ron was the youngest of their three boys, born many years after the others.

Initially, this gentle, articulate young man who presented with a good scholastic record, a well-developed sense of humor, and compassion for other patients, responded well to psychotropic medication and intensive staff support. Six weeks later he was discharged with an Axis I diagnosis of Brief Reactive Psychosis (American Psychiatric Association, 1987).

During the next four years, Ron was admitted to the same psychiatric unit of the community hospital six times. Each admission was precipitated by a dramatic psychotic episode. For example, although he was able to finish a bachelor's degree in business administration, he could not find a suitable job. By his own account, he lost the jobs during the interviews. When his father became hospitalized for a mild coronary infarction, he stopped the job search to help his mother with household chores. His own words are most expressive. "I was putting the groceries into the car when I saw the message flashing at me, you know, on the grocery bags there is a little square of writing at the center on the top? It was flashing "help your father." I took a deep breath and looked away. When I looked back, it was still flashing the message and I thought, "oh no, it's happening again." He left the bags in the shopping cart and went to a florist where he bought a dozen roses. A few hours later he personally delivered them to the psychiatric unit. By this time he was responding to auditory commands warning him to fulfill his mission to mankind. During this hospitalization, Ron's psychic disorganization became apparent. Euphoria over his special "calling" alternated with fright. After two months, he was discharged with symptoms under control but with evidence of grandiosity and expansiveness in his thought content. Now the discharge diagnosis on Axis I was Schizophrenia, Undifferentiated Type, subchronic with acute exacerbation (American Psychiatric Association, 1987). The global assessment of functioning had dropped from a level of 82 when he first consulted a psychiatrist to 44. Plans were made for Ron to receive outpatient therapy and medication follow-up at the hospital clinic.

A different admission was precipitated by bursts of frenzied, disorganized activity including an uncharacteristic preoccupation with sports events. He was working as a bookkeeper in a local department store, a position that he believed to be far below his abilities. One warm day he came home at noon carrying a basketball. His mother was sitting in a lawn chair. He stood behind her and began bouncing the basketball on her head. She said, "stop that, Ron." He said "I can't, Ma. You'd better get me to the hospital before I really hurt you." Again there were several weeks of hospitalization before symptoms were controlled enough for release.

On this admission, with his endocrine system demonstrating adverse reactions to neuroleptic treatment, medications were temporarily discontinued. Now, disturbing visual hallucinations complicated his interactions with staff. For example, when asked why he would not make eye contact with a trusted staff member he replied, "I know you wouldn't do this to me, but when you smile, fangs dripping blood come out of your mouth." On another occasion he stared at the wall behind the staff member who was talking with him. When asked if he were looking at something on the wall (which was blank) he replied, "I'm watching those eyes on the wall." A different medication was tried and eventually symptoms were controlled, but a definite blunting of affect was observed. Ron's normally articulate speech was sprinkled with loose associations.

The prognosis for maintaining an independent life outside of a special facility was guarded. Ron's father had taken early retirement and his mother was concerned as to the effects of Ron's erratic behavior on his father's health. She also admitted to being afraid of Ron. Without much comment, Ron accepted the suggestion that he go to a half-way house in the community. He managed there for a number of months with outpatient follow-up and a brief admission following the onset of insulin-dependent Diabetes.

Ron begged his family to take him home. Seeking some family support and connection in their retirement, his parents had sold their home to move closer to his brother's family. Reluctantly, they agreed to a trial visit. A few days before his scheduled return to the half-way house, Ron did not appear for breakfast. Since staying up most of the night and then sleeping late had been his pattern on this visit, no one checked on him until noon. Ron could not be roused. By the time the ambulance arrived, vital signs had ceased. The cause of death was attributed to complications of diabetes. After four years, Ron's nightmare was over.

Vignette #2

Rachael was an intelligent, high-spirited third-year psychology major who maintained good grades, a work study position at the college and a part-time career singing with a local rock group. Until her mother was admitted to the psychiatric service of the hospital, Rachael successfully concealed the reason she avoided making friends who might expect to be invited into her house.

Rachael had been the acting head of the household for the six years since her father's death. Life insurance policies, plus Social Security provided a limited financial income for the family. Over the years, her mother who retreated more and more into her bedroom, was treated by the family doctor for what the children were told was a "nervous condition." According to Rachael, it was not until her own illness began and her uncle told her that she "was just like her mother," that relatives revealed that the post-partum episodes required her mother to be hospitalized for months after the birth of each child.

Rachael presented for help at the College Counseling Center. Resources were mobilized through the collaboration of Center staff with the Social Service Department of the hospital where Rachael's mother was a patient. It was eventually determined, with Rachael's input, that her mother needed placement in a long-term care facility. Rachael continued to receive counseling at the college through the school year. Although Rachael was functioning at a high level, she was still the head of the family. As part of their termination, the college counselor arranged for Rachael to continue support in a group conducted by an area psychologist at a reduced fee.

Exactly one year after her mother's hospital admission, Rachael decided to drop out of school. Recent incidents such as her sister's automobile accident, financial problems with reimbursement for her mother's care, and her brother's school problems seemed realistic stressors. She had stopped attending group sessions some weeks earlier, and now she was behind in school work. The private psychologist reported that he had scheduled three appointments which she had failed to keep. The psychologist was interested in working with Rachael in individual sessions, but she was no longer returning his calls.

During a meeting with the same female counselor that she had seen the year before, Rachael expressed feelings of abandonment at the transfer to the psychologist. When the counselor related the psychologist's concern for her, Rachael said she did not believe a man could relate to her situation. She told the counselor she could only work with her. Rachael's former enthusiasm had been replaced by an agitated intensity, intermingled with expressions of despair. Two days later, she formally withdrew from school. On that weekend, she ingested a number of Valium left over from her mother's supply. She was admitted via the emergency room to the same psychiatric unit where her mother had been one year before.

Except for a sedative at bedtime, no medications were prescribed. Rachael responded rapidly to the staff and the therapeutic milieu. As the agitation calmed, a more depressive affect emerged. She described her reason for taking the Valium as "just being overwhelmed." After five weeks, the discharge diagnosis was Adjustment disorder with depressed mood (American Psychiatric Association, 1987). Discharge plans were to return to school for spring semester and to resume counseling at the college with her former counselor. When the counselor expressed some concerns with this arrangement, it was modified to include a visit with the psychiatrist once a month. In the counseling sessions, Rachael seemed to pick up where she'd left off eight months before; however, she started to arrive very early for her session, often ahead of the student with the appointment before hers. She began dropping into the center at unappointed times, bringing the counselor unrequested coffee or lunch. When attempts to explore the meaning of this behavior were evaded, the counselor set firm limits to which Rachael responded with flirtatious, then angry remarks.

Again the sessions ended for the summer. Rachael, who was already one semester behind, failed to complete the work for three of the five courses in which she was enrolled, virtually assuring that she would be in the university for one more year. During the summer break, only one session a month was scheduled at the counseling center; the psychiatrist would also continue his once monthly visit. During one of the appointmentless weeks, Rachael arrived uninvited at the counselor's home. She had obtained the address through a work-study student in an administrative office on the pretense that she had it already but had misplaced it. She talked with the baby-sitter, met the children and waited for the counselor to return. When the counselor asked her to leave, stating that the visit was inappropriate and would be discussed at the next scheduled session, Rachael became visibly distressed. She pleaded to be allowed to stay for dinner, offering to help with the children. Although the counselor was firm, Rachael began a flirtatious teasing and did not depart for another half hour. Again, at the next session, she dismissed the behavior as "no big deal."

During the fall semester, Rachael began to express doubts about having placed her mother in a long-term facility. Rachael began to speculate that the counselor had forced her decision. Shortly after, she went away for a hiking week-end with some people she had met in class. She returned early, reporting angry fights with the others whom she saw as selfish. Again, she pondered dropping out of school. When the counselor reminded her that their sessions were contingent upon her being a student, she responded, "oh, I know I can get you to see me anyway. Besides, I've been thinking about moving out of my house and asking you if I can be your live-in baby-sitter." When the counselor began exploring that notion as a fantasy, Rachael got angry and refused to discuss it. She dropped out of school before completing the semester. She took a job as a nurse's aide, stopped seeing the psychiatrist and called the counselor several times a day, at first at work and then during the night, begging her to let her move in. Rachael's younger sisters brought her to the emergency room after she had gathered some clothes in the center of the living room and set them on fire.

During this psychiatric admission, the hypothesis of learned behavior from her mother was discarded. Rachael's agitation required medication. She expressed both suicidal ideation and hostility toward the counselor, who she believed had rejected her. She was both hostile and manipulative with staff, finally getting them to persuade the counselor to come to the psychiatric unit for a joint session. Rachael was elated. Although the counselor told Rachael that she needed the special skills of the psychiatrist instead of her, Rachael dismissed this, saying "I always know that in the end I'll get what I want from people." When it was apparent that she would not get to resume her relationship with the counselor, Rachael became enraged, aggressive and assaultive and had to be sedated and secluded. Following these outbursts, she became profoundly depressed. After four months, she was released from the unit, to be followed up at the community mental health center. Her discharge diagnosis at this time was Borderline Personality Disorder (American Psychiatric Association, 1987). In the 12 years since that discharge, Rachael has had at least 10 hospital admissions, ranging in duration from a few weeks to more than a year. Some of these admissions were precipitated by suicide attempts, and some followed psychotic episodes that have publicly threatened others. On another occasion, the police were required to remove her from the Counseling Center of the College, where she had camped out, disheveled and carrying a baseball bat, vowing to remain until someone told her where her former counselor was now working. She became assaultive and abusive and was again admitted for psychiatric help.

Rachael is known to every mental health facility within a 25-mile radius. Her diagnoses have included Manic (bipolar) disorder, Multiple Personality disorder, and Erotomanic delusional (paranoid) disorder (American Psychiatric Association, 1987). Her medical history reads like a chronicle of psychiatric medications, treatments, and supportive and alternative therapies common to the latter part of the 20th century. And despite involvement with numerous counselors and therapists representative of all the professions engaged in mental health work, she continues, 12 years later, to harass her first counselor in many creative and disruptive ways.

Rachael's mother died about 10 years ago. Because of the unpredictable and threatening behavior associated with her transient psychotic episodes, she has not lived with her siblings for many years. Only her youngest brother maintains any contact with her. Now her primary residence alternates between the state psychiatric hospital and various community half-way or group homes. Although she did manage to complete requirements for a bachelor's degree in psychology, Rachael has not had any continuous employment since the nurse's aide job more than a decade ago. She is occupied full time by her mental illness.

Use of the Trajectory Model of Nursing in Multiple Sclerosis

Suzanne C. Smeltzer, R.N., C., Ed.D.

College of Allied Health Sciences
Thomas Jefferson University
Philadelphia, PA

Multiple sclerosis (MS) is a chronic, demyelinating disorder that is unpredictable in its overall course, in the type of symptoms that will predominate, and in its eventual outcome. It has been used as a model in research, education, and practice to examine the course of chronic illness, patient and family responses, coping and adjustment to chronic illness, and specific concepts and variables of interest to researchers. MS is used in this paper to evaluate for nursing practice the utility of the Corbin and Strauss trajectory model of nursing. The assumptions and major concepts of the trajectory framework are discussed, use of the model in multiple sclerosis is demonstrated, and the strengths and limitations of the framework as a nursing model are identified.

MS has been used repeatedly in research as a model of chronic illness to examine the course of chronic illness and those services required during its various phases, to examine patient and family responses, coping, and adjustment, and to examine specific concepts and variables of interest to researchers including uncertainty, hardiness, and social support (Pollock, Christian, & Sands, 1990; Wineman, 1990; Larsen, 1990). Those characteristics that make MS useful as a model of chronic illness—its uncertainty and unpredictability and its progressive and disabling qualities—make it difficult for patients and their families to predict its course and plan their lives. It is often equally difficult for health care providers to identify appropriate medical and nursing interventions, given the unpredictable course that the disease may take. The trajectory framework has the potential to guide nursing practice when the patient or client has MS. This paper provides a description of MS, identifies the assumptions and major concepts of the trajectory framework, and applies the framework specifically to MS. Strengths and limitations of the framework as a nursing model are also identified.

DESCRIPTION OF MS

MS is an acquired demyelinating disease of the central nervous system character-ized by wide variability in its symptoms and in its course. It is one of the most common diseases capable of producing severe disability in young adults. The age of onset is usually between 20 and 45 years of age, with a mean age at onset of 33 years. MS can, however, occur at virtually any age. Its cause is unknown, and no definitive therapy yet exists to alter its course (Cook, 1990).

Contrary to the perceptions of many health care providers, MS is not inevitably a terminal disease, and severe disability does not occur in all cases of MS. Despite the image of MS as a disease that will result in all patients being wheelchair-bound or bedridden in a few short years, the course of the disease may range across a wide spectrum. Although most patients have a course that is characterized by remis-sions and exacerbations with or without progression, other disease courses are possible. Some patients do have a rapid downhill course and early disability, while others have a subclinical course with the diagnosis made only on incidental magnetic resonance imaging (MRI) brain scan or at autopsy (Cook, 1990). More typically, MS follows a course somewhere between these two extremes. At least 20% of patients experience the *benign* form which is characterized by sensory disturbances. Despite years of illness, no significant disability usually results, and patients with this form generally have a normal life span. Twenty-five percent of patients have the *relapsing-remitting* (exacerbating-remitting) form of the dis-ease, with attacks that often leave little residual disability. Those with the relapsing-remitting form of MS tend to have fewer attacks over time. The *relapsing-progressive* type, seen in 40% of patients, is similar to the relapsing-remitting form, but the patient does not return to baseline, and progressive disability occurs. There may be acute fluctuations superimposed on a progressive course. A smaller number of patients (15%) experience slowly progressive deficits over time without remissions or exacerbations. The disease may begin as the relapsing-remitting form and become *chronic progressive* later. Once a course has become progressive, return to a remitting course is unlikely. Five to ten percent of patients may have a *malignant* or rapid downhill course (Smith & Scheinberg, 1990).

In most cases, the initial attack of MS resolves completely, or nearly so, and the patient remains well until the next attack. Onset of attacks may be acute or abrupt; in other patients, the symptoms of an exacerbation are slow to appear, taking several days to develop. Remission of symptoms tends to occur within weeks to a few months. Once progression has begun, it generally continues, but at a relatively slow rate. Even in patients with a more progressive course, the disease may appear to stabilize for long periods of time. The wide variations in the possible disease course, or trajectory, make it unpredictable and uncertain. Although the course of the disease over the first five years provides a clue, on a statistical basis, to the subsequent progression, it is difficult, if not impossible, to predict the disease course on an individual basis.

Wide variations in the possible manifestations of MS also exist. Clinical manifestations range from sensory symptoms that can be bothersome and annoying (e.g., numbness, tingling, burning, or tightness) to those that can be distracting and intolerable (e.g., persistent burning, discomfort or pain syndromes). Other symptoms may include gait disturbance and ataxia, bowel, bladder, and sexual dysfunction, and muscle weakness, spasm, and spasticity. Lesions in the brain stem may produce nystagmus, impaired ocular motility, and dysarthria; impaired vision is not uncommon. Memory loss and cognitive difficulty of varying degrees may also occur. Fatigue may be very disabling and may interfere with the patient's ability to work or participate in family and social life. Although there is considerable variation in the possible symptoms of MS, it is uncommon for all manifestations to occur in every patient (Miller, 1990).

The diagnosis of MS and the ability to assess effectiveness of treatments are also characterized by uncertainty; until recently, the diagnosis was made through the process of elimination of other disorders that could be responsible for the constellation of symptoms. The newer methods of diagnosis available today, including MRI, do not provide definitive proof that MS is the cause of symptoms; furthermore, clinical symptoms are often not correlated with the results of diagnostic tests (Smith & Scheinberg, 1990). The waxing and waning of symptoms that often occur with MS make it difficult to evaluate the effectiveness of different medical treatments or nursing interventions because one may be unable to categorically attribute improvement of symptoms, a slowing in progression of the disease or improvement in overall health status or well being to treatment effects, patient's actions or the natural course of the disease. In summary, MS is unpredictable in its overall course, in the occurrence of the next attack, in the type of symptoms that will predominate, in its eventual outcome, in its diagnosis, and in evaluation of therapies.

THE TRAJECTORY FRAMEWORK AS A NURSING MODEL

Trajectory Framework

The trajectory framework is derived from the science of sociology via the grounded theory method. The original purpose of the trajectory approach was to gain greater understanding of what it is like to live with, cope with, and manage a chronic illness. The major concept underlying the model of chronic illness presented by Corbin and Strauss is the trajectory of the illness course; it is described as the concept that unites other conceptualizations of the framework. The trajectory framework is based on the premises that chronic illnesses have a course that varies and changes over time, and that the illness course can be shaped and managed even if the course of the disease itself cannot be modified. The purposes of the framework then are: (a) to change the course of disease, prevent its downward spiral or delay or slow the progression of symptoms, and (b) to manage signs, symptoms, and problems that occur and to maintain quality of life (Strauss, et al., 1984). The explicit and implicit assumptions underlying the trajectory model include: (a) the chronic illness course can be shaped (explicit assumption); (b) knowledge of the patient's trajectory perception of illness will assist in shaping or managing its course (explicit assumption); and, (c) the chronic illness trajectory is ultimately a downward spiral (implicit assumption implied by the definition of trajectory).

Functions of a Nursing Model

To be useful as a model of nursing, the framework must serve as a general guideline for nursing practice, research, teaching, and administration. In the practice setting, a model assists in identifying what data are important to observe, formulating nursing diagnoses, and directing nursing interventions. It guides assessment strategies and provides guidelines about interpretation of assessment data, the design of nursing interventions, and direction for outcome criteria for evaluation (Fawcett, 1984).

Nursing's Metaparadigm in the Trajectory Framework

The four metaparadigm concepts of nursing—person, health, environment, and nursing—are explicitly defined and discussed by Corbin and Strauss in their discussion of the trajectory framework as a model for nursing. Person is defined within the trajectory model as an individual who has a chronic illness; goals are to prevent chronic illness or manage it if it is not preventable, while maintaining a high quality of life. The person's biography and events of everyday life are aspects of life that go on despite the illness, but also influence the chronic illness trajectory. The patient and family are identified as primary and active participants in the prevention of complications and management of illness. The explicit definition of health, identified in the trajectory framework, is presented from an illness perspective. Health is described implicitly, however, in terms of Smith's (1983) category of the adaptive model of health, which incorporates concern about the patient's role performance and ability to respond to and cope effectively with change. The patient's home is identified as the primary environment because it is the site of most of the patient's activities including management of the chronic condition. High technology and transition from one environment (home) to another (hospital or rehabilitation center) are explicitly defined as part of the patient's environment. Within the trajectory model, nursing is defined as supportive assistance directed toward the individual patient, family, community, and society. Nursing functions range from provision of complex care to counseling and monitoring. These functions are congruent with the view of the patient as the primary participant and director of his or her own management. Although not explicitly stated, the points at which these concepts intercept create the setting for nursing action. The trajectory framework includes characteristics from several types of conceptual models of nursing, including systems models and interaction models; if one considers the phases and subphases of the illness trajectory as a process of development, the trajectory framework could be described as a developmental model.

In the nurse's interaction with patients with a disorder such as MS, the trajectory framework would focus attention on the patient's perception of the illness and on assessment of those factors that influence the patient's and family's ability to manage and deal with the consequences of the disease and its unpredictable course. It would encourage consideration of factors that promote adaptation and coping with the disorder and identification of those factors that impede that adaptation process. The trajectory framework focuses on the everyday activity and life work and their effect on management of a chronic illness. Additionally, it emphasizes the teaching, counseling, directing, and coordinating roles of the nurse that nurses consider so fundamental to their practice.

Application of Trajectory Framework to MS

In MS, the goals of many newly diagnosed patients and their families and those health care providers with a cure orientation are to change the course of disease, prevent its downward spiral, and arrest the disease progression. Often it is only in the absence of a cure that the goal of management of problems associated with the illness and maintaining and improving the quality of life becomes acceptable to the patient and family and many health care providers. Use of the trajectory model has the potential to bring much needed focus and attention to this latter goal. With MS, this rarely means keeping the patient comfortable and free of complications for a few months or years until death; more often it means maintaining the highest level of physical and psychological health and well-being possible throughout the course of the illness, a course that may last for 50 years or longer. Therefore, use of the trajectory model to identify and explore the course of the patient's illness and strategies to deal with the chronic disorder has the potential for an enormous positive impact on this goal.

Corbin and Strauss define trajectory projection as one's vision or perception of the illness course; it encompasses the meaning of the illness, its symptoms, its biography, and time. All those who come in contact with the illness and its management are assumed to have their own vision of the course of the illness and ideas about how it can and should be shaped. While knowledge of the trajectory projection will assist an affected individual, family, and health care providers to plan for the future and cope with the chronic illness, the unpredictable and varying course and symptoms of some chronic illnesses, specifically MS, may result in different projections among patient, family, and health care providers (Strauss et al., 1984). The trajectory projections of the patient and family are often influenced by the views, beliefs, opinions, and responses of their health care providers. Because many health care providers often have continued contact only with those persons whose course of MS is progressive or severely disabling, their projection of the trajectory of MS is often that MS will inevitably result in the patient's early death after years of being bedridden. Those with a less severe course may not seek health care regularly; therefore health care providers, including nurses, may have little experience with those individuals who have only occasional MS symptoms or relapses but between attacks are able to participate fully in all family, work, and social activities.

Patients report being told by many health care providers that nothing can be done to alter the disease course, "there is nothing further we can do for you," a view that emanates partly from an orientation toward cure and partly from lack of information about the many variations in the course of MS. These views may be inconsistent with the ultimate pattern of exacerbations and remissions and the true disease course. Life plans may be altered based on projections that the disease trajectory is always severe and disabling. Patients may make important decisions on the basis of projected trajectories that never materialize. For example, a young woman with a new diagnosis of MS may forgo marriage and childbearing because of others' persuasive views that she will eventually be bedridden, that MS will be made worse by pregnancy, and that she will be unable to care for her children or live long enough to see them grow up. Years later she may find that the MS course was benign or not severely debilitating and unlikely to have had any effect on childbearing after all (Smeltzer, in review). Mishel (1988) has suggested that uncertainty may have positive effects when it permits hope that the illness is not as severe as feared. Uncertainty may allow the patient and family to retain hope, while a feeling of certainty that one is very likely to be severely disabled based on trajectory projections of others may remove all possibility of hope.

The trajectory projection influences interventions and attitudes and motivates patients, their families, and the physician or nurse to take action when symptoms appear or additional problems develop. The expectation that the disorder will result in potential shortening of the life span of the affected individual may influence and alter family interactions (Benoliel, 1983). Belief that MS complications and disability are inevitable may hamper the patient's efforts to continue participation in life's activities. If health care providers believe that all MS patients will ultimately develop complications such as aspiration or pneumonia, they are not likely to be concerned with identifying and reducing the risks of these life-threatening complications (Smeltzer, Lavietes, Troiano, & Cook, 1989; Smeltzer, Utell, Rudick, & Herndon, 1988). Patients may ignore decrements in function or well-being if they believe that long-term complications such as urinary incontinence are inevitable. Although many MS symptoms cannot be reversed or prevented, many can be managed; however, others may never even occur.

Differences in trajectory projections of patients and their families may lead to differences in their management goals (Corbin & Strauss, 1984). When the views of patients and family members differ from those of the patient's health care providers, the possible consequences include unmet expectations and dissatisfaction (Thorne & Robinson, 1988). While patients and their families may consider the primary goal to be reducing the effects of MS and promoting as normal a life as possible, this may conflict with the goal of a health care provider whose focus is cure. Failure of health care providers to explore and respond to the patient's trajectory projection may avoid giving the patient an accurate picture of the eventual illness course, but it leaves the patient susceptible to vague, inaccurate or misguided advice from other sources, e.g., "rest," "decrease the stress in your life," "don't ever get pregnant" (Smeltzer, in review). Patients and their family members often move from one health care provider to another to find one whose views are more congruent with their own (Strauss et al., 1984). Although projection of the illness' trajectory is a key issue in the model, the consequences of different trajectory projections on the management of MS and its symptoms and on the relationships of involved individuals are not fully addressed in the trajectory framework (Thorne & Robinson, 1988; Yarcheski, 1988). However, identification of the trajectory projections of those involved in the management of the illness, is certainly a necessary first step to addressing this issue.

THE TRAJECTORY FRAMEWORK AS A NURSING MODEL IN MS

To be useful for clinical nursing practice, the trajectory model must be specific enough to address any chronic disease and general enough to provide direction for practice. Therefore, the four steps used by Corbin and Strauss to demonstrate use of the framework in nursing will be discussed to demonstrate how it might be applied to this chronic illness.

Step 1: Locating the Client and Family and Setting Goals

The first step in using the trajectory framework in nursing practice is assessing and locating the patient along three dimensions of the trajectory—illness, biography, and everyday life activities—and examining any interactive effects among them.

Illness. An important aspect of assessment is exploring the course of the patient's MS and pattern of symptoms to date in order to anticipate patient goals. Only if the patient's current health status is known and is compared to past health status (for example, six weeks, six months or six years ago), can the nurse get a sense for the trajectory of the illness and the patient's projection of its trajectory. This assessment is essential if the nurse is to work with the patient to identify goals for management of current problems and formulation of goals for the future. The patient's current activity level and the level of functioning aspired to are important for assisting the patient in reaching those goals. It is important to determine what the patient and family understand about MS, as they may have heard MS referred to as "the great crippler of young adults..." Their knowledge may be influenced by worst-case scenarios that are reported to them by well-meaning friends.

There is little doubt that, if given a choice of preventing MS or learning to live with it, individuals with MS would want to prevent its occurrence or arrest its progression. However, since this is not possible, the goal becomes keeping the illness under control and minimizing its effects on the patient's and family's lives. This goal depends in part on the extent and nature of MS symptoms, the disease course, and the view of the patient and family about how controllable or treatable the MS symptoms and possible complications are. If the MS course is one punctuated by occasional attacks but a return to a normal level of function after each attack, the patient's goal may be learning to deal with its uncertainty and unpredictability. If the MS course is one in which disability occurs progressively or sporadically, prevention of complications and management of disability are likely goals and major responsibilities of the patient and family.

The visibility of the illness to others may affect the patient's and family's ability to deal with the chronic illness (Benoliel, 1983). If a disorder has high social visibility, that is, it is obvious to laypersons, the patient and family are often unable to disguise or hide it. Consequently, if a person with MS experiences muscle weakness and balance problems that result in use of a wheelchair, that individual may not be expected to explain decreased participation in work, social, and family activities and the reasons for changes in the roles of family members. On the other hand, the MS patient with disabling fatigue, who does not appear sick, and his other family members may find themselves asked about changes in their usual roles when the patient is unable to fulfill society's expectations for making a living or caring for children.

Assessment of the trajectory scheme includes exploring the patient's response to the appearance of new MS symptoms. Patients often attribute to MS every symptom they ever experience, including those that cannot be attributed to MS; the symptoms' appearance may produce anxiety in the patient and fear that the MS is progressing. During an exacerbation, the patient may "hold his or her breath" to see if the symptoms will abate this time or what degree of disability will remain following the attack. Other persons with MS are symptom-responsive; that is, they often respond to symptoms between exacerbations by seeking treatment, but between attacks they may forgo health care. Until or unless there is some interference with activities or the occurrence of frightening, potentially threatening symptoms (e.g., decreased vision, increasing muscle weakness), they may pay no attention to MS. The patient may not consider herself to have a chronic illness, especially if completely symptom-free between exacerbations.

Biography. Identification of the patient's approaches to treatment and use of strategies to prevent exacerbations or progression of MS or to manage symptoms can provide insight into the patient's methods of coping with MS and implications for future management. The type of therapy (traditional vs. nontraditional; experimental vs. nonexperimental therapies), the number of various clinical trials the patient has participated in, and the lengths to which the patient has gone in an effort to obtain relief or "cure" may provide some insight into the patient's coming to terms with MS. If a patient continues to seek cure through unproven, nontraditional or perhaps harmful therapies, he or she may be ignoring significant problems associated with MS in the hope that they will be remedied by some future miracle therapy. Additionally, the patient may not attend to other aspects of life while searching for a cure. While cure is not the focus of nursing, the patient must be allowed to continue to hope for a cure while simultaneously learning to prevent complications, to maximize quality of life, and to find ways to manage and live with MS. "Coming to terms" with MS is the process of making the modifications that are necessary in order to live with its consequences. Often, repeated adjustments must be made as the illness course changes. Other patients may elect not to undergo either traditional treatments or newer or promising experimental therapies because of disturbing side effects, lack of faith in health care providers and the health care system, or fear that they may run out of treatment options in the future when they "may really need it."

Everyday Life Activities. These activities include those actions of daily living through which persons live out the many aspects of the self. Assessing the impact of MS on the patient's identity and every day life activities provides information about the patient's expectations and goals. This includes assessing the changes in the patient's life and those of the family because of MS symptoms. The role of the nurse will be different when working with a patient who retires from former activities because of interference by severe disability, one who retires because of anticipation of future disability, and the wheelchair-bound patient who puts in a full work week or who finds an alternative way to engage in work, family, and social activities.

Patients and their families often are expected to assume major responsibility for management of symptoms and complications while trying to continue relationships and carry on ordinary experiences of living (Benoliel, 1983; Corbin & Strauss, 1984). They are expected to maintain "normal" lives and to experience and deal with the usual developmental human and family life experiences that are part of everyone's existence. MS produces not only a series of changes for the affected individual, but also has the potential to affect family relationships. The appearance of MS may initiate a reorganization of family structure and style; the family structure, in turn, may undergo modifications as new phases of the illness appear. Disorganizing effects of chronic disease tend to appear whenever there is a major change in the family life cycle (Benoliel, 1983). Shifts in family life cycle may in turn affect the management of the chronic disease. For example, in MS these disorganizing effects become evident when a mother with MS who has young children is hospitalized for a short course of immunosuppressive therapy or when a teenager who has played a major role in helping his affected parent deal with some aspects of the chronic illness prepares to go away to college. These same effects are likely to occur with every change in the phases or subphases of the illness or every family stage. Without assessment and exploration of these shifts and changes in family organization and relationships during patient and family contact with the health care system, patients with MS and their families are unassisted and left to their own devices.

Chronicity requires a continuous state of modification and revision as the individual moves from status to status through the experience of the human life cycle (Benoliel, 1983). The father with MS who has young children may have to revise his expectations about what activities he is able to share with them. The need of the person with MS to change occupations or cease working completely because of symptoms of MS may affect the roles of the patient and spouse in their relationship. In order to provide her young child with physical activities that she is unable to provide, a mother may enroll her child in a play group or nursery school earlier than she ordinarily would have planned; as her children grow older, the MS symptoms may progress and further limit her ability to participate in their activities. The woman with progressive MS may have to choose between participation in a successful career and staying home with her children because her fatigue level does not permit her to balance both activities in her life. The elderly husband may be unable to continue lifting his wife with MS from the bed to a chair because his chest pain has recently been diagnosed as angina.

Limitations management is part of everyday life activities and refers to the alterations and adaptations necessitated by the person to permit carrying out those activities. In MS, limitations management may include avoiding activities that bring on symptoms or make living with symptoms difficult, e.g., avoiding activities in the afternoon when fatigue in MS tends to be greatest, limiting activity when increased symptoms occur, resting when the children are napping so that the patient can rest but still be able to take care of the children, or planning the day so that the stairs have to be climbed only once. In more progressive or disabling forms of MS, these strategies might include making arrangements with others to assist with eating, daily hygiene, or transportation to see health care providers.

Examination of the interaction of the chronic illness, biography, and performance of everyday life activities provides information about their combined impact. Only if one understands the patience and careful planning that are necessary for successful management of MS can the nurse or other health care provider be of assistance to patients and families as they acquire new strategies to deal with changes and increasing disability that occur with progressive forms of the disease while living as normal a life as possible.

Step 2: Assessing Conditions Influencing Management

Identifying those factors that facilitate or interfere with the ability of the patient and family to manage the MS trajectory and achieve their goals is important because it identifies those variables that often can be manipulated to reach those goals. Those conditions that influence the patient's and family's ability to manage the course of MS may include resources (e.g., time, money, energy, manpower, equipment, technology, and knowledge), social support, the presence of other health problems in the family, and past experience with management of MS, as well as other health problems. The presence and extent of cognitive changes secondary to MS must be identified, as they may influence the ability of the patient to understand and follow through with instructions and procedures that may be needed in managing the trajectory of MS. Information about the lifestyles of the patient and family, their goals and aspirations, and the nature of the interactions of the patient and family are assessed, as they influence management strategies. An understanding of the economic and political issues that bear upon management is essential if the nurse is to assist the patient and family to identify and obtain the maximum supports available. This is particularly important when the course of MS is progressive and further deterioration of physical functioning is anticipated.

Patients with chronic illness and their families have often developed a high degree of expertise in management of symptoms and disabilities. Staff are frequently not knowledgeable about the patient's MS symptoms, responses to MS, or the effects of MS on the lives of the patient and family. The ability of the patient and family to manage the disease course effectively and to achieve and make significant contributions to the lives of others despite MS is often not recognized or acknowledged by health care providers (Thorne & Robinson, 1988). Hospital staff frequently do not explore the effect and meaning of hospitalization to the MS patient and family. Hospitalization may be perceived as a crisis. It may be considered to signify: 1) deterioration of the patient's condition or progression of the disease; 2) failure to manage illness or disability adequately; 3) vulnerability to the actions of others; or 4) risk that the patient's and family's skills and expertise in management will be ignored or disregarded. If the patient is hospitalized with non-MS problems, concerns related to MS may be ignored or all problems may be attributed to MS (Smeltzer, in review). Little if any discussion of MS-related issues and concerns may take place because of fear on the part of health care providers that bringing up issues may depress, disturb, or otherwise upset the patient. Assessment of these aspects is essential if one is to understand the patient's responses and concerns as well as those of the family.

The home, where most of the day-to-day activities of the person with MS take place, needs to be assessed to determine if home arrangements promote or impede the patient's ability to live as normal a life as possible. It is in the home where patients fulfill their various roles. Because women are more commonly affected with MS than men, the impact of MS on their roles as spouse, mother, caretaker, and breadwinner if they become more symptomatic and disabled, and the importance of each of those roles to them will influence the amount of the time and energy available for management of the chronic illness. The patient and family may not think about simple household modifications, e.g., installation of grab bars in the bathroom and elevation of the toilet seat, that can improve the patient's ability to function independently. Patients and their family members may not consider more extensive renovations (e.g., installing a concrete ramp to the house to accommodate a wheelchair, widening doors) because of expense. The impact of modifications that affect other members of the household (e.g., moving a bed into the living room if a patient is unable to climb steps to a second floor bedroom) and their acceptability to the patient as well as the family must be assessed. The costs of these modifications and the availability of family, community, and state funds to assist financially with such modifications often determine whether they will be implemented and reduce the social isolation experienced by the patient. The patient and family must also be psychologically ready for these alterations and the meaning of their necessity and permanence.

High technology is generally not associated with MS except in the area of ambulatory assistive devices (e.g., motorized wheelchair), and treatments themselves do not appear dramatic, as do dialysis machines or ventilators. Because management of MS rarely requires highly technical equipment and all the additional assistance that seems to follow such treatment, those persons with MS must be prepared to be active participants in management.

Step 3: Defining the Intervention Focus

This stage refers to defining the target of intervention to determine what should be manipulated or modified to enable the patient to reach desired goals. If it is obvious that the patient, family, and health care provider hold different views about the MS trajectory, it is important to identify the impact of these differences on its management. Additionally, if the primary goal of the patient is to obtain a cure for MS, it is necessary to assist the patient and family to manage the disease trajectory and prevent complications while preserving their hope for a cure in the future. The patient and family must be given information about the current phase of the illness trajectory, with specific information to enable them to deal with current problems while anticipating and planning appropriately for the future. Failure to identify and address the long term needs of MS patients is often a result of ignorance about the natural history of the disorder and an ingrained feeling of hopelessness about its outcomes. Many MS patients tend to be labeled by health care providers as having the more severe and progressive form of the disease even before such a pattern has become evident (Maloney, 1985). Generalizations about MS may lead to loss of hope on the part of the patient and family or expectations that are unrealistically high or low.

Step 4: Intervention

The focus of nursing in MS is not on cure but on the patient's and family's living with and shaping the disease course and preventing complications while promoting and maintaining their quality of life through supportive assistance. The occurrence of attacks of MS and progression of the disease manifestations are usually out of the hands of the patient, family, and health care provider; that is, they do not depend on the patient's adherence to regular treatment modalities or prevention strategies, as do insulin administration, dialysis treatments, or dietary modification. The prevention of complications and minimization of the effects of disability, however, are often under the control of the patient and family. To enable patients and families to be active participants and coordinators of care, they must have enough information for informed decision making. Nursing intervention in MS requires that the nurse collaborate with the patient and family, recognizing their critical role in management and as members of the multidisciplinary team, not merely as the passive recipients of care from others. Additionally, the nurse must collaborate closely with other health care providers to offer appropriate care and support to the patient and family. Prevention of MS complications, continuity of care, and management strategies occur within the context of the specific characteristics of the patient's MS symptoms and overall illness trajectory, its treatment, and the patient's personal biography and daily activities. When the patient with MS is hospitalized, efforts must be taken to assure that the patient maintains as much control of care as desired, while simultaneously allowing the patient and family to obtain respite. Because of increased symptoms or increased fatigue, the patient who is hospitalized with an exacerbation may be unable to carry on normal activities. The patient must, however, be the director of what is needed and wanted in the way of assistance. The patient must be treated as the adult and responsible person whose wishes for self-care must be honored even if they are not within the usual hospital schedule or protocol.

Step 5: Evaluating the Effectiveness

Because of the trajectory of MS, it is difficult to establish clear-cut or objective criteria to evaluate the effectiveness of interventions. The effects of interventions on the ability of the patient and family to manage the illness course and prevent complications, and to maintain a quality of life that is acceptable for the patient and family are goals that are consistent with the trajectory framework. The input of the patient with MS and his or her family in the identification of evaluative criteria is important if they are to exercise their roles as important members of the management team. If evaluation criteria are established independently of patient and family input, it is unlikely that those criteria will be met. Only if evaluation strategies are flexible and responsive to changes in the patient's trajectory, life cycle, and ability to manage and adapt, will evaluation keep pace with and reflect those changes.

CRITIQUE OF THE TRAJECTORY FRAMEWORK
AS A MODEL FOR NURSING

As is evident from use of the trajectory framework as a model for nursing in MS, the framework encourages the nurse to consider the patient holistically, with consideration of the patient's and family's critical roles in management of the chronic illness. Its focus on those factors that influence management of the course of chronic illness increases the potential impact of nursing on health care and the quality of life of the person with MS. The strength of the framework as a model for nursing is clearly demonstrated in the first two steps of the process: (a) locating the client and family and setting goals and (b) assessing conditions influencing management. Previously published reports (Corbin & Strauss, 1984, 1985; Strauss & Glaser, 1975; Strauss et al., 1984) have clearly demonstrated insight and understanding of the strategies used by patients and their families to cope with and manage chronic illnesses. Less obvious, however, is the role that is advocated by the trajectory model for health care providers, particularly nurses, when patients and families are the major participants in illness management and the primary directors of care. The emphasis on assessment and understanding of the impact of chronic illness on the patient and family may be the best evidence and support for the view that the nurse's interventions will be directed largely by the patient and family. Supportive assistance, which includes teaching, counseling, monitoring, and coordinating roles, is recognized for its importance in assisting the patient and family in their management of the chronic illness.

Little direction is provided by the framework for nursing interventions in those circumstances where the disease trajectory is very uncertain. Although it is clear that the trajectory model can be applied with ease to management of the MS trajectory in the patient whose disease is progressive or physically disabling to any degree, it is less obvious how the model can be used to address the illness trajectory of those patients who are symptom-free for long periods of time between attacks. To consider as chronically ill the patient diagnosed with a chronic illness such as MS but who may be without symptoms for many years may negatively affect the patient's overall attitude and lifestyle. Those persons with MS and other chronic illnesses that are characterized by long, symptom-free periods may not establish routines to manage their illness and may not seek resources to assist them because their illness courses are too unpredictable. While transition from wellness to illness states has received considerable attention from researchers, little attention has been given to the transition from an illness to wellness state (Davis, 1987); such a transition may characterize the patient with a relapsing-remitting disease such as MS, who experiences complete remission of symptoms between attacks. The focus of the trajectory framework on chronic illness as a process in time, rather than as a single point in time, implies movement of the patient through a sequence of stages or steps (Meleis, 1991). Consequently it promotes insight into the behaviors of the MS patient and family during exacerbations as well as between exacerbations when the patient elects to ignore the disease and concentrate on living rather than on being chronically ill. Using the trajectory framework, management issues that are often of major importance in a cure orientation or medical model approach to management (e.g., strict compliance to rigid therapeutic regimens), take a position secondary to life management issues if the patient is to live a full life despite MS as opposed to allowing MS to become his life. Further guidance from the framework is needed for these circumstances.

Many important concepts presented in earlier work (Strauss & Glaser, 1975; Strauss et al., 1984), such as managing regimens, reordering time, etc., are not identified and discussed as part of the trajectory nursing model. Although a conceptual model may provide general direction for nursing practice, the nurse who utilizes the trajectory model as a framework for practice must become familiar with the theory that has emerged from the trajectory model of chronicity. Because one can gain insight into and understanding of chronicity by following and studying patients and their families as they manage the chronic illnesses, longitudinal research methods and case studies seem warranted. For the nurse to grasp the complexities faced by the chronically ill patient and his or her family, strategies to enable the nursing student or nurse in practice, even in an acute care setting, to follow chronically ill patients over time could be explored. Further description of the concepts considered critical to the metaparadigm of nursing (Fawcett, 1984) is needed if the trajectory framework is to gain further acceptance in nursing; more explicit definition of these concepts would clarify the category of conceptual model considered by the authors to fit the trajectory framework.

Despite these limitations, the trajectory framework holds great potential and promise for nursing; because of the increase in the number of persons affected by chronic illness, use of the trajectory model would allow nurses to make significant contributions to the lives of chronically ill patients and their families. Only by examining the course of the patient's illness over time and gaining insight into the effects of chronic illness on the life of patient and family can nurses even begin to make a difference. Because the trajectory framework is not limited to a single discipline and is appropriate for all settings where those with chronic illness can be found, it will allow and encourage collaboration among members of health care disciplines and promote care that crosses the boundaries of home, hospital, office, clinic, and long-term care facility.

REFERENCES

Benoliel, J. Q. (1983). Grounded theory and qualitative data: The socializing influences of life-threatening disease on identity development. In Wooldridge, P. J., Schmitt, M. H., Skipper, J. K., & Leonard, R. C., *Behavioral science and nursing theory* (pp. 141-187). St. Louis: C. V. Mosby.

Cook, S. D. (1990). *Handbook of multiple sclerosis.* New York: Marcel Dekker, Inc.

Corbin, J. M., & Strauss, A. L. (1984). Collaboration: Couples working together to manage chronic illness. *Image: Journal of Nursing Scholarship, 16*, 109-115.

Corbin, J. M., & Strauss, A. L. (1985). Managing chronic illness at home: Three lines of work. *Qualitative Sociology*, 224-247.

Davis, L. L. (1987). Convalescence and implications for nursing research. *Image: Journal of Nursing Scholarship, 19*, 117–120.

Fawcett, J. (1984). *Analysis and evaluation of conceptual models of nursing*. Philadelphia: F. A. Davis.

Larsen, P. D. (1990). Psychosocial adjustment in multiple sclerosis. *Rehabilitation Nursing, 15*, 242–246.

Maloney, F. P. (1985). Rehabilitation of patients with progressive and remitting disorders. In Maloney, F. P., Burks, J. S., Ringel, S. P., *Interdisciplinary rehabilitation of multiple sclerosis and neuromuscular disorders*. Philadelphia: J. B. Lippincott.

Meleis, A. I. (1991). *Theoretical nursing: Development and progress*. Philadelphia: J. B. Lippincott.

Miller, A. E. (1990). Clinical Features. In Cook, S. D. (Ed). *Handbook of multiple sclerosis*. New York: Marcel Dekker, Inc.

Mishel, M. H. (1988). Uncertainty in illness. *Image: Journal of Nursing Scholarship, 20*, 225-232.

Pollock, S. E., Christian, B. J., & Sands, D. (1990). Responses to chronic illness: Analysis of psychological and physiological adaptation. *Nursing Research, 39*, 300–304.

Smeltzer, S.C., (1991). Concerns of pregnant women with Multiple Sclerosis. Unpublished manuscript

Smeltzer, S. C., Utell, M. J., Rudick, R. A., & Herndon, R. M. (1988). Pulmonary function and dysfunction in multiple sclerosis. *Archives of Neurology, 45*, 1245–1249.

Smeltzer, S. C., Lavietes, M. H., Troiano, R., & Cook, S. D. (1989). Testing of an index of pulmonary dysfunction in multiple sclerosis. *Nursing Research, 38*, 370–374.

Smith, C. R., & Scheinberg, L. (1990). Symptomatic treatment and rehabilitation. In Cook, S. D. (Ed.), *Handbook of multiple sclerosis*. New York: Marcel Decker, Inc.

Smith, J. A. (1983). *The idea of health: Implications for the nursing professional*. New York: Teachers College, Columbia University Press.

Strauss, A. L., & Glaser, B. G. (1975). *Chronic illness and the quality of life* (1st Edition). St. Louis: C. V. Mosby.

Strauss, A. L., Corbin, J., Fagerhaugh, S., Glaser, B. G., Maines, D., Suczek, B., & Wiener, C. L. (1984). *Chronic illness and the quality of life* (2nd Edition). St. Louis: C. V. Mosby.

Thorne, S. E., & Robinson, C. A. (1988). Health care relationships: The chronic illness perspective. *Research in Nursing and Health, 11*, 293–300.

Wineman, N. M. (1990). Adaptation to multiple sclerosis: The role of social support, functional disability, and perceived uncertainty. *Nursing Research, 39*, 294–299.

Yarcheski, A. (1988). Uncertainty in illness and the future. *Western Journal of Nursing Research, 10*, 401–413.

Shaping the Course of a Marathon: Using the Trajectory Framework for Diabetes Mellitus

Elizabeth A. Walker, R.N., D.N.Sc.

The Diabetes Research and Training Center
Albert Einstein College of Medicine
Bronx, New York

Persons with either insulin-dependent or non-insulin-dependent diabetes mellitus live with a chronic illness that can have both acute and long-term complications. The therapeutic regimen for glycemic control in diabetes is often complex and is lifelong; it requires special knowledge and skills for both patients and health care providers. In this article, the Corbin and Strauss trajectory framework for chronic illness management is clinically applied to the planning of patient care in two case studies of persons with diabetes. The benefits of using the trajectory framework as a model for care in diabetes include: introduction of the concepts of "locating" the patient on the trajectory and assessing the trajectory projection for both patient and provider, and a more realistic evaluation of incremental change in chronic illness. Two possible barriers to clinical application of the framework for diabetes management are: difficulty in translating the framework for clinical use, and some terminology in the framework that does not seem to describe reimbursable care. The trajectory framework provides a necessary shift in focus to quality of life issues in diabetes management over the lifespan.

Application of the Corbin and Strauss trajectory framework to build a model for nursing care for the person with diabetes appears, at first glance, to be a simple task. The purpose of this response, however, is to move through the "first glance" to attempt specific clinical application of the major concepts of the framework, and to describe perceived benefits of and barriers to using the trajectory framework for diabetes nursing care.

Diabetes mellitus encompasses a group of genetically heterogenous chronic disorders which are characterized by abnormalities in carbohydrate, protein, and fat metabolism; the common denominator is hyperglycemia (Rifkin & Porte, 1990). Prolonged hyperglycemia is a toxic condition which can produce both microvascular and macrovasular damage over time. Two major clinical subclasses of this disorder are insulin-dependent diabetes mellitus (IDDM), known as type I diabetes, and non-insulin-dependent diabetes mellitus (NIDDM), or type II diabetes (Sperling, 1988). Both types of diabetes are chronic disorders, but their etiology, clinical presentation, acute complications, and course of illness can be quite dissimilar.

The acute complications of diabetes include severe hyperglycemia, resulting in diabetic ketoacidosis or hyperosmolar nonketotic coma, and profound hypoglycemia. Chronic or long-term complications of diabetes are generally the result of macrovascular, microvascular, or neurologic pathologies. Persons with diabetes face increased risk of cardiovascular disease, with greater incidence of myocardial infarction, hypertension, and lipid abnormalities. Neuropathies can occur as distal polyneuropathies or autonomic neuropathies such as impotence and orthostatic hypotension. Persons with diabetes are 25 times more at risk for retinopathy leading to blindness than the general population. Nephropathy, leading to end-stage renal disease, and lower extremity amputation are complications for which persons with diabetes are at increased risk (Centers for Disease Control, 1990).

Minimizing the acute complications and avoiding or delaying the chronic complications of diabetes are often the major goals of therapy. Depending on the type of diabetes, there are various levels of complexity for a therapeutic regimen to meet these goals (Lebovitz, 1988). Patient adherence to the complex regimen for control of blood glucose is one of the more problematic aspects of diabetes care. Both health provider and patient may have the knowledge and skills to control blood glucose. But patients, with their support systems, have to enact this knowledge in their daily routines without, at present, any guarantee that control of their blood glucose will decrease their risk of developing chronic complications. The Diabetes Complications and Control Trial (DCCT) is a prospective, multi-center, national study designed to answer this question about the relationship between blood glucose control and development of complications for insulin-dependent diabetes (The DCCT Research Group, 1987).

Caring for persons with diabetes, especially in the outpatient setting, is regarded by health care providers as the initiation of a lengthy therapeutic relationship. As Metz (1988) described: "the *sine qua non* of good diabetes therapy is to persuade, encourage, coach, and equip patients to develop the knowledge, tenacity, courage, and optimism necessary for long-term successful management of their diabetes" (p. 3). It is in fact "their" diabetes, and it is alternately described as an illness or wellness ("I just have trouble with my blood sugars"); as a burden or a blessing ("My whole family eats healthier foods now"); and as the health provider's problem ("Why don't you make me exercise?") or theirs ("Just leave me alone!"). Thus, enhancing patients' motivation to continue performing the complex daily regimen is the challenge to health providers, for "...the diabetic person's race is no sprint; it is more than a marathon" (Pichert, 1986, p. 97).

CLINICAL APPLICATION

Two patient cases are presented to assist in the clinical application of the trajectory framework for advanced nursing practice in the specialty of diabetes management.

Cyrus is a 28-year-old, slender, white male with insulin-dependent diabetes mellitus (IDDM) of 11 years duration. The first four years after diagnosis were marked by his resistance to following the insulin and dietary recommendations given to him. He had multiple episodes of severe hypoglycemia and two hospitalizations for ketoacidosis. He graduated from college at age 24, and was married and became a father that same year. At his wife's insistence, he had an appointment with a specialist in a diabetes team practice. Cyrus admits that he now wishes to get control of his diabetes. He has recently experienced several episodes of hypoglycemia without the usual warning symptoms; during one of these episodes his wife reported that he seemed to be having a seizure. A final problem which he briefly mentions is that his wife desires a second child; he, however, is having "some trouble with sex."

Maria is a 55-year-old, obese Hispanic woman with newly diagnosed non-insulin-dependent diabetes mellitus (NIDDM). After her husband died, she applied for a job to help support her two teenage children. Her fasting blood glucose was 190 mg/dl when she had her employment physical. Even though several of her relatives have diabetes, she had not had her blood glucose checked in 12 years. When she visits the city-supported medical clinic, her chief complaints are fatigue, numbness in her feet, and blurry vision at times. Her blood pressure is 150/98, and she has a small amount of protein in her urine. Maria states that she is overwhelmed by the amount of change in her life subsequent to her husband's death.

The nurse in advanced practice managing care for Cyrus in a diabetes team setting, or for Maria in a clinic setting is challenged to individualize a therapeutic regimen which has some hope of success in terms of metabolic control, patient adherence, and quality of life (Anderson, Nowacek, & Richards, 1988). The concepts of the Corbin and Strauss trajectory framework are used to build an advanced nursing model for diabetes management.

In "locating" Cyrus at Step 1 of a trajectory-based nursing process, the nurse elicits a complete nursing history including: his trajectory scheme, trajectory projection, his present trajectory phase, and everyday activities of his regimen for diabetes. The nurse requests specific information concerning his reported hypoglycemia unawareness, possible seizure, and "trouble with sex." The nurse would also incorporate the results of the medical history and physical, including laboratory indices of metabolic control (e.g., blood glucose, lipids, hemoglobin Alc [HbAlc]). Complete locating of Cyrus could not be accomplished during this first visit, and goal setting with this patient would have to be quite broad at this point. Patients generally need to know what it takes in terms of behavior changes before agreeing to specific goals, such as decreasing the HbA1c by 2% or limiting the total fat in their diet to less than 30% of their calories.

Cyrus may agree that he is now in an "unstable trajectory phase;" he may be ready to initiate some change in his "trajectory scheme" in order to become more stable. Parts of both Step 2 (assessing the conditions influencing management) and Step 3 (defining the intervention) would need to occur next. For example, general goals may be to avoid hypoglycemia and seizure and to stabilize Cyrus' blood glucose levels. The nurse as part of the treatment team may discuss with Cyrus the possibility of taking multiple injections of regular insulin with a long-acting insulin each day, rather than his present regimen of one injection of NPH and regular insulin in the morning. Changing to this scheme would also involve frequent blood glucose monitoring, perhaps three to four times each day. Both of these changes involve economic resources, insurance coverage for supplies, increased complexity of the regimen, and lifestyle changes. Thus, in order to establish mutual realistic goals (Step 1), the nurse and patient must consider elements of Steps 2 and 3.

Two concepts in the trajectory framework of particular interest for Cyrus are trajectory projection and reciprocal impact. How Cyrus views the course of his chronic illness, his trajectory projection, would provide invaluable information for managed care. For example, he was a teenager when he was diagnosed. Does he now have a mature understanding of diabetes? Does he view himself as ill or well in an acute and chronic sense? Is he optimistic about the future or does he see himself as a blind amputee on dialysis by age 40? How does he view his current problems? Has he lost control of his blood glucose and his sexual function?

The reciprocal impact of intensifying insulin therapy for Cyrus must be considered. Although he was experiencing insulin reactions, his average blood glucose control was poor, with a HbA1c of 14% (Tanenberg, Alster, & Tuttleman, 1990). Increased injections of insulin to more closely mimic the pancreas must be accompanied for patient safety by frequent self-monitoring of blood glucose. Changes in diet and exercise may also be considered as part of the intensified treatment. Thus, many lifestyle changes would have to be incorporated into this new regimen. If the reciprocal impact of all these changes is assessed by either Cyrus or the nurse as too great, perhaps there could be a scheme for achieving incremental, planned change over time. Keeping in mind the analogy of the course of diabetes being a marathon and not a sprint is helpful at times. Because Cyrus is being treated in a diabetes team setting, coordination and evaluation of the intervention among the various team members (endocrinologist, dietitian, nurse specialist) will be particularly important responsibilities of the nurse managing his care. Quality of life, metabolic control, patient adherence, and appropriateness and complexity of the regimen must be continually reassessed.

Maria, a patient at a city-supported medical clinic, is newly diagnosed with non-insulin-dependent diabetes (NIDDM) . The concept of projectory phasing is particularly important for nursing care in NIDDM because of the usual uncertainty of the date of onset of this illness. There can be a prolonged asymptomatic phase before actual diagnosis (Centers for Disease Control, 1990). Maria has already reported at the time of her diagnosis the numbness in her lower extremities, usually considered a chronic complication of diabetes. Thus, Maria has rapidly moved through the phases of pretrajectory, onset, and perhaps into an unstable phase, considering also her blurry vision and neuropathic feet.

The nurse planning interventions with this newly widowed patient could benefit from the assessment structure of many key concepts of the trajectory model, e.g., trajectory projection, conditions influencing management, biographical and everyday living impact, and a projection of the reciprocal impact of a therapeutic regimen for progress toward control of at least her blood glucose, with some weight loss. This patient's view of the illness course for diabetes could easily be colored by the history of other family members who were known to have had diabetes. These histories could range from a sister who had a myocardial infarction at age 50 to an uncle who "never took care of his diabetes" and lived a productive life to age 80. Family histories often provide conflicting messages about the trajectory projection for persons with diabetes.

The health provider's vision of Maria's illness trajectory is also an important self-assessment. Maria may already have some neuropathy; there is reason to screen further for nephropathy, retinopathy, and hypertension. The nurse could view Maria's course as in a downward phase; this patient may be seen as too overwhelming an educational or counseling task for this busy clinic setting, where each patient visit is allotted only 15 minutes. The required lifestyle changes may include a low-fat, low-protein, and lower calorie diet for this Hispanic, obese, middle-aged woman. The concept of trajectory projection for this patient and her health provider draws attention to possible underlying affective responses to this new diagnosis and proposed treatments; these affective responses must be dealt with in order to create an optimal management plan with this patient, with proper outside referrals and support.

BENEFITS AND BARRIERS

There are significant benefits of using the trajectory framework to build a nursing care model for diabetes. First, the focus of this framework is the chronicity of an illness. In a busy health care setting, often the acute hypoglycemic or hyperglycemic events of diabetics are attended to, while the plan to decrease risks of the chronic events may be left undone for lack of reflective time for the provider. Locating patients in terms of their trajectory phases, keeping in mind the timing over years of greater risk for each chronic complication, would be invaluable for comprehensive care planning, especially in a multidisciplinary team conference.

Second, the concepts of this framework useful for assessing the patient with diabetes (e.g., trajectory projection, biographical and everyday living impact, reciprocal impact) provide a rich source of data for mutual goal setting and care planning. These data can be used well for developing the often complex therapeutic regimens that require many lifestyle changes. Since a major goal in this framework is quality of life, the health provider is reminded to assess this factor at each step of the process. Utilizing trajectory phases (e.g., a downward phase of decreased adherence) is also an appropriate way to assess that a patient may need permission to "take a vacation" from an intense regimen for a specified period of time. For example, a patient who wears an insulin pump and self-monitors his blood glucose four times a day may wish to switch to two insulin injections a day for a brief period of time in order to decrease the impact on everyday living, i.e., the complexity, of his chronic illness.

A final benefit of using a framework developed for chronicity is that the evaluation phase is put into proper perspective. Progress toward change is often undervalued, as it is less quantifiable than a dramatic change in lifestyle behaviors or metabolic control. It is this progress, however, that may lead to long-term incorporation of exercise, stress management, or proper nutrition into daily living. Consider a patient who has been counseled about incorporating regular exercise (e.g., 30 minutes, three times each week) into a weekly regimen. After six weeks when the patient reports that there have been only five minutes of planned exercise managed each week, the provider's response may be optimistic ("She has made a small change"), or pessimistic ("Forget exercise!") (Seligman, 1991). Small, incremental change can, perhaps, be recognized and appreciated with optimism within this framework for long-term behavior change in chronic illness.

There are several barriers to successful utilization of this framework. For clinical application, the translation of a framework must be clear. A graphic view of the framework for clarification of relationships between concepts is a necessity for the health provider. Strauss and Corbin (1990, p.221) presented such a diagram in their recently published qualitative research book. This rather complex diagram, however, would require yet further translation prior to becoming useful for a nursing model. By necessity, with the course of a chronic illness, the diagram will be complex; but this complexity begs for an easily translatable guide to be understood not only by nurses, but also by physicians, dietitians, and other members of the health team who care for persons with diabetes.

Another barrier to successful use of the trajectory framework for advanced nursing practice in diabetes is that the terminology does not always sound reimbursable. For example, nursing management, counseling, and education in diabetes are labor-intensive processes, usually performed in the outpatient setting. Convincing third-party payers from the insurance industry and the government that what a nurse does is necessary, beneficial, and cost-effective has continued to be a major reimbursement problem. Terminology from the trajectory framework, such as "supportive assistance" and "arrangement-making," are descriptive of important functions, and they may be helpful in teaching, and perhaps research, of these concepts. For clinical practice, however, these terms do not project an image of skilled nursing care and would probably be avoided when describing rationale for direct reimbursement for nursing services. Third-party reimbursement for what is termed "patient education" continues to be a major challenge in many states; patient education has at times been referred to as "skills counseling for self-management" in order to increase the chances of reimbursement for this nursing care. Thus, the labels for nursing care are important, and some of the terminology of the trajectory framework may be a barrier to reimbursement for these very necessary clinical nursing activities.

CONCLUSIONS

As portrayed by the case studies of Cyrus and Maria, IDDM and NIDDM are two distinct chronic illnesses that are called diabetes. Managed care for these patients can be overwhelming, and, at times, the priorities for the major therapeutic goals get confused. Are we focusing on metabolic control, adherence to the regimen, or quality of life? Are we attending more to the acute rather than the chronic complications? If 10 years of hyperglycemia have passed without planned care, it may be too late to decrease the risks of microvascular and macrovascular complications.

The trajectory framework provides excellent concepts for developing a model for education in advanced nursing practice for chronic illness. Descriptive research of these concepts could provide rich data for understanding the multifactorial nature of patient nonadherence to complex therapeutic regimens. Clinical nursing practice may well benefit from a model based on this framework; the benefits derived would increase greatly if the trajectory concepts and relationships could be easily translated for multidisciplinary care planning. Shaping the course of illness and wellness for the person with diabetes, utilizing the trajectory framework, would provide a depth and breadth to advanced nursing practice in diabetes.

REFERENCES

Anderson, R., Nowacek, G., & Richards, F. (1988). Influencing the personal meaning of diabetes: Research and practice. *Diabetes Educator, 14,* 297-302.

Centers for Disease Control (1990). *The prevention and treatment of complications of diabetes.* Atlanta, GA: Department of Health and Human Services.

Lebovitz, H. (Ed.) (1988). *Physician's guide to noninsulin-dependent (type II) diabetes.* Alexandria, VA: American Diabetes Association.

Metz, R. (1988). Overture: The patient and the provider. In R. Metz & J. Benson (Eds.), *Management and education of the diabetic patient* (pp. 3-9). Philadelphia, PA: W. B. Saunders.

Pichert, J. (1986). But I want to motivate you. *The Diabetes Educator, 12,* 96-97.

Rifkin, H. & Porte, D. (Eds.) (1990). *Diabetes mellitus: Theory and practice* (4th ed.). New York: Esevier.

Seligman, M. (1991). *Learned optimism*. New York: Alfred A. Knopf, Inc.

Sperling, M. (Ed.) (1988). *The physician's guide to insulin-dependent (type I) diabetes.* Alexandria, VA: American Diabetes Association.

Strauss, A. & Corbin, J. (1990). *Basics of qualitative research: Grounded theory procedures and techniques.* Newbury Park, CA: Sage Publications.

Tanenberg, R., Alster, D. & Tuttleman, M. (1990). Diabetes mellitus. In T. Moore & R.C. Eastman (Eds.), *Diagnostic endocrinology* (pp. 167-182). Philadelphia: B.D. Decker, Inc.

The DCCT Research Group (1987). Diabetes Complications and Control Trial (DCCT): Results of the feasibility study. *Diabetes Care, 10,* 1-19.

Acknowledgment. This work was supported by the Diabetes Research and Training Center, Albert Einstein College of Medicine, Grant # DK20541

Commentary

We begin this brief commentary with two expressions of appreciation. The first is to the Editors of the *Scholarly Inquiry* journal, whose innovative format stimulated genuine, thoughtful, and intensely focused dialogue among the several authors about significant aspects of chronic illness and nursing care. We also deeply appreciate the time, energy, and reflection devoted by the six authors invited to assess the trajectory model for its potential usefulness in their own areas of expertise.

In general, those assessments are strongly positive. There is little point for us to highlight the reasons for this—readers will see and judge for themselves. Rather we shall (a) attempt to clear up occasional misunderstandings about the trajectory model, (b) touch on a few suggestions made in criticism or supplementation of the model, and (c) say a few words in answer to the one author who strongly criticized the model.

THE MISUNDERSTANDINGS

First. The course of illness is not inevitably downward. A large proportion of chronic illnesses does involve physical deterioration, but not inevitably. They may stabilize, especially those that need proper management and get it. Some illnesses are relatively stable, though they may have downward phases that soon or eventually stabilize at original levels of functioning.

Second. Chronic illnesses do not necessarily end in death. A great proportion of them do not, and some may not if properly managed.

Third. Another occasional misunderstanding is that "trajectory" refers only to the illness course itself. A closer look at the definition and discussion should make it clear that the action "around" the illness course, especially the attempts to shape it, is an essential part of the concept of trajectory.

Fourth. Generally the authors have understood that the model offers only general guidelines, and that, in the words of one author (Elizabeth Walker), it is necessary "to attempt to build specific clinical applications of the major concepts of this [trajectory] framework." This was one of our central points, but sometimes it gets either overlooked or forgotten, with the consequence that the model is inappropriately criticized for failing to account for some important aspect of the *particular* chronic illness under discussion. There was also a tendency to overlook the emphasis on the prevention aspects that is part of the trajectory model.

BARRIERS AND ELABORATIONS

Those misunderstandings are the source of a few of the criticisms made of the model, and these we will not address. The remaining criticisms are more in the nature of thoughtful points raised about barriers to the model's usefulness or suggestions for elaborating on it. For instance, "some of the terminology of the trajectory framework may be a barrier to reimbursement for...very necessary clinical nursing activities.... The terminology does not always sound reimbursable" (Elizabeth Walker). This point is, of course, part of a more general problem of conveying to third-party payers "that what a nurse does is necessary, beneficial, and cost effective." We agree that the model seems not to address this problem of persuasion, but why can't inventive nurses alter some of the terminology for purposes of persuasion? Yet it is important to have recognized this issue. The same author notes that for the health provider, "some more graphic translation of the model is necessary." She may well be right, at least for some readers.

Another author (Suzanne Smeltzer) finds that in the model, "Many important concepts presented in earlier work, such as managing regimen, have been omitted; therefore, "the nurse who utilizes the trajectory model as a framework for practice must become familiar with the theory that has [already] emerged from the trajectory model of chronicity." Smeltzer is right about the first point. About her second point, we do not believe that practitioners necessarily need to be familiar with the previous work or theory associated with the model, but certainly the work of those who use it in research or teaching would profit directly from knowing those materials.

We were pleased to see that several good ideas concerning questions or directions for research were suggested by the reading of our paper. Another kind of suggestion—one with which we strongly agree—concerned the need for educating nurses with regard to particular chronic illnesses in directions pointed to by the trajectory model. We read also with particular interest Mary Hawthorne's passages about the impact of new and changing medical technology on both the staffs themselves (underlining acute rather than chronic care functions) and on the production of new phases of old trajectories (for instance, the "chronically critically ill"). This interplay of technology and chronic illness is very important to understand, whether the technology consists of equipment, drugs, tests, or even the procedures of "soft technology." As some readers will recognize, we wrote about some of this interplay in a previous publication by Strauss, Fagerhaugh, Suczek, and Wiener (1985), *The Social Organization of Medical Work*, but it is good to have it brought up to date, and specifically for this highly technologized area of chronic illness. It may be useful here to quote a few lines from something written by the same authors about these new phases.

In our study of medical work in hospitals, we were struck by a new phenomenon: the effectiveness of contemporary medical technology and medical/nursing procedures in making it possible for people to live with chronic illnesses from which they would previously have died. This does not mean that the survivors are always physically comfortable or without grave symptomatology. The more usual pattern is that new developments in the illness, as well as new symptoms, appear. With time, clinicians learn to handle these new symptoms, by using, for example, new drugs that were developed for this purpose. Alas, these too may produce 'side effects' that perhaps will require additional drugs or other technologies to manage, and so on. Such new phases of illness frequently call for multiple therapies (cancer therapies are an example). And then, the chronically ill often have multiple illnesses—each illness perhaps moving into previously unknown phases.

Because the trajectory model is based on studies or observations of chronic illnesses, including those discussed by the other authors, in reading these papers, we have not been surprised by the general tenor of their assessments. Occasionally, however, while reading the papers we were much surprised and delighted at particular ideas that had never occurred to us. The most striking instance was Marilyn Rawnsley's conclusion that use of the trajectory model might not only "signal an exciting 'comeback' of professional and public interest in promoting quality of life" for the mentally ill but also "lead to a 'restoration' of respect" for the mental health professionals themselves.

Kathleen Nokes' thoughtful report on the usefulness of the trajectory framework when applied to AIDS has fortified our own impressions with regard to this illness—at first understandably conceived of as deadly but recognized now as increasingly a chronic illness in the industrialized countries where treatment is available. One of us (Strauss) and his research team has been studying AIDS policy and has written a paper (1991) detailing how AIDS is highlighting a series of deficiencies, or gaps, in the health care system. They include those in: home care, equity, care offered the homeless, care offered addicts, and deficiencies in managing new trajectory phases.

AIDS is also having enormous impact on economic aspects of health care, as well as raising profound moral issues. Basically, this chronic illness highlights many of the economic and moral issues attending chronic illness in general: what weight to give personal responsibility and societal responsibility. Central, too, are questions of expenditures and cost containment. Also, on whom should limited health dollars be spent? Such decisions involve balancing questions of equity against national efficiency and rewards for individual attainment in a relatively open society.

Even more basically,"every industrialized nation is facing how to manage—financially as well as medically and humanly—the increasing rate of chronic disabilities. These are being generated both by conditions of life in contemporary societies and by the dramatically increasing longevity of their citizens. Our own population has opted for high-tech medicine, combined with a patchwork ... of types of health services." Understandably, AIDS is putting additional stress on that patchwork.

THE DISSENTING ASSESSMENT

There was one strongly critical assessment by Diane Scott Dorsett, who rejects the trajectory model. She finds it completely inadequate for the care (and the lives) of cancer patients who are either in remission or cured. She classifies the trajectory model as really a variant of the "illness-medical paradigm," as contrasted with a "recovery trajectory framework." She proposes that "the *course of recovery* is a more relevant trajectory for cancer as a specific chronic disease and as a general framework for clinical science." The emphasis of this competing framework is on possible recovery or actual physical cure ("the survival picture has changed, resulting in many more prolonged remissions and, in many cases, cure").

This is hardly an appropriate place for a full debate on these issues. We will confine ourselves to a few points that "accentuate the positive" rather than the negative, except to point out in passing that Diane Scott Dorsett misreads a number of aspects of our presentation along the lines suggested earlier under Misunderstandings, and these are central to her criticisms of the trajectory model. Readers will surely catch the many misreadings of our paper, and even those of the 1975 edition of *Chronic Illness and the Quality of Life* (the unrevised edition) that Scott Dorsett seems to have used as a supplementary reference on trajectory. More important, her misreadings have perhaps blinded her to possibly fruitful ways of combining overlapping features of the two models.

Perhaps the best way to reconcile the two models' features is as follows. With some varieties of cancer disease there are, of course, increasingly long periods of remission. These are not stable trajectory phases in the usual sense that the illness has to be carefully managed in order to keep it from getting worse. People who are in cancer remissions do have to be monitored for changes of physical conditions, but otherwise little or no medical treatment is required. This is another instance where the recent technologies have resulted in a type of new trajectory phase.

By "new phase" we mean, again, that an illness condition had not been seen previously, or at least was seen infrequently, if it occurred spontaneously without medical intervention. Also, the range of management actions occurring in terms of the remissions, especially the long ones referred to by Scott Dorsett, has changed in tandem with the new physiological conditions. For every emergent new trajectory phase, medical and nursing staffs (and kin) have to learn the appropriate steps to work out the most effective caring procedures. So these new trajectory phases, which we see evolving for many chronic illnesses today, constitute very important new elements of the chronic illness scene. It follows that whenever particular chronic illnesses and their associated technologies are producing new phases, the latter should receive specific names; the naming would tend to focus attention on the new phenomena and so promote better care, research, and education during these phases.

Some of the most urgent drama attending new trajectory phases, as with cardiac disease, takes place in the ICU, with its consequent emphasis on acute versus chronic conditions. In other illnesses, the major drama can take place both in or at the health facilities (chemotherapy) and/or at home (struggling with the effects of chemotherapy, or psychologically "working through" anxieties about whether a "remission" will be permanent).

The literature, as well as our own observations, suggests that people with cancer who are going through remissions, however long these may be, are unlikely simply to think of themselves as cured "forever." Recurrent or permanent anxiety is characteristic of a remission trajectory phase when potential or possible death lies at its end. As for cancer patients who are actually "cured"—if they really are, then are we talking about a chronic illness or a cured one?

Not to cavil, however, we read Scott Dorsett's recovery trajectory framework as a worthy effort to bring patients back into their own management and to give them hope and encouragement and psychological techniques for managing their lives. Providing that nurses do this without ever forgetting that people with cancer have experienced suffering, have identities that bear the scars of struggle, and that these must enter into the new phases of their remission (even "cured") trajectories, then we would agree that a "recovery" model is something that can be combined with our own model. Taken in that sense, we do not see them as competing. What worries us a bit is that nurses in practice may overlook or minimize the biographical/identity aspects of patients in an effort to promote courage and "realism"—with a kind of cheerfulness that might be, if not rejected as callous, at least rejected as "not understanding me." Worse yet, if a patient is dying or preparing to die, he or she needs psychological closure on life, the staunchly recovery-committed nurse is unlikely to be of much help with that vital process of "coming to [final] terms."

In short, we are emphasizing that a central feature of *any* chronic illness, unless the symptoms are really nonintrusive, is that people have to *live* with those illnesses, i.e., come to terms with them and the symptoms, their regimens, and whatever side effects of the regimens that may appear. Helping them to live with their illnesses, symptoms, side effects, and the impact of these on their identities and their life styles, is part of the work of their kin, their significant others, and health professionals. If aspects of the recovery model can help, especially with persons whose actual illness courses warrant helping to build optimism or fortitude or some psychological reactions in the direction of "recovery"—if they can help, then we applaud this direction of nursing care and the model that encourages it. In this sense, we believe the two models are overlapping. In other ways, of course, they are not.

THE TRAJECTORY MODEL: NEXT STEPS

What is needed next with respect to this model? We suggest the following. Perhaps it does not so much need "testing" as further clarification, elaboration, and qualification (where parts of it do not fit well with or omit features of particular illness or illness conditions). These ends can be reached, presumably, through several paths. A first path: innovative practice using the model, and critical judgments about where it works well and where not. A second: using the model, research into other chronic illnesses; also research into new emergent trajectory phases; and research into particular phases or aspects of already studied illnesses, but now in greater depth. A third path: clarification of the model's concepts and their relationships, as well as the careful clarification of additional concepts that will evolve from the practice and research paths. Think then of this model as only a beginning, albeit one that has been used for some years in research and in students' and ex-students' practices. Presumably, too, it is only one of several models that we need to develop for today's prevalent types of illness, those that are presently chronic.

REFERENCES

Strauss, A., Fagerhaugh, S., Suczek, B., & Wiener, C. (1985). *The social organization of medical work.* Chicago: University of Chicago.
Strauss, A., Fagerhaugh, S., Suczek, B., & Wiener, C. (1991, July). AIDS and health care deficiencies. *Society,* page numbers unavailable at time of publication.
Strauss, A., & Glaser, B. (1975) *Chronic illness and the quality of life.* St. Louis: Mosby. (Revised edition, 1984, by A. Strauss, J. Corbin, S. Fagerhaugh, B. Glaser, D. Maines, and C. Wiener.)

Juliet Corbin
Anselm Strauss